The Carnivore Diet

Special Edition - Two Books

Carnivore Diet With Intermittent Fasting. Combine Two Powerful Strategies For Rapid Fat Loss and Increased Health

Michael D. Kaiser

The Carnivore Diet

The Carnivore Diet with Intermittent Fasting - Combine Two Powerful Strategies For Rapid Fat Loss and Increased Health

Special Edition – Two Books

© Copyright 2019 – Michael D. Kaiser
All rights reserved

Published by:

CyberLearners, LLC.
Cleveland, Ohio

Legal Disclaimer

The follow book is reproduced below with the goal of providing information that is as accurate and reliable as possible. Regardless, purchasing this book can be seen as consent to the fact that both the publisher and the author of this book are in no way experts on the topics discussed within and that any recommendations or suggestions that are made herein are for entertainment purposes only. Professionals should be consulted as needed prior to undertaking any of the action endorsed herein.

This declaration is deemed fair and valid by both the American Bar Association and the Committee of Publishers Association and is legally binding throughout the United States.

Furthermore, the transmission, duplication or reproduction of any of the following work including specific information will be considered an illegal act irrespective of if it is done electronically or in print. This extends to creating a secondary or tertiary copy of the work or a recorded copy and is only allowed with express written consent from the Publisher. All additional right reserved.

The information in the following pages is broadly considered to be a truthful and accurate account of facts and as such any inattention, use or misuse of the information in question by the reader will render any resulting actions solely under their purview. There are no scenarios in which the publisher or the original author of this work can be in any fashion deemed liable for any hardship or damages that may befall them after undertaking information described herein.

Additionally, the information in the following pages is intended only for informational purposes and should thus be thought of as universal. As befitting its nature, it is presented without assurance regarding its prolonged validity or interim quality. Trademarks that are mentioned are done without written consent and can in no way be considered an endorsement from the trademark holder.

This book is not giving medical advice.

Book One

The Carnivore Diet

Eat Meat to Quickly Lose Fat, Lean Out and Cleanse Your Body.

Includes Meal Plans to Get You Started Today

Michael D Kaiser

Receive free alerts for Carnivore Diet meal plans and testimonials

www.CarnivoreCleanse.com

Table of Contents

Chapter One: What is the Carnivore Diet? 10

Chapter Two: The History of the Carnivore Diet 17

Chapter Three: Getting Started with the Carnivore Diet 27

Chapter Four: The Three Levels of the Carnivore Diet 37

Chapter Five: Best Meals for the Carnivore Diet..................... 49

Chapter Six: Benefits of the Carnivore Diet............................. 82

References 87

Introduction

This book is based on someone that decided to try the Carnivore Diet plan after not being able to burn off the remaining sub-cutaneous layer of fat, even though he was exercising intensely, lifting weights, doing fasting and high intensity training, eating clean and healthy, etc.

When the author tried the meat only diet for 7 days, he was very afraid of health repercussions or developing high cholesterol. But NONE of that happened, in fact his cholesterol went down 7 points and his energy ZOOMED, and his abs finally showed after only 7 days, plus working out routinely as well. Previously he was on a mostly vegan diet. The author decided that the carnivore diet is really great for resetting the body metabolism and health, almost like a cleanse if you want to use that term.

There are great benefits to eating whole plant-based foods, but for some people it is not enough; if you are one of these people, the Carnivore Diet may be great for you to reset or even switch over to long term. The key is to eat only WHOLE meats, not processed meats.

The following chapters will discuss the carnivore diet and everything that it entails. Like most people, you probably do not think it is possible to survive, thrive and receive health benefits on a meat-only diet. Yet there are numerous people doing exactly that.

There are numerous instances in history when civilizations survived on nothing else but meat diets only. There are numerous studies from around the world that showcase how communities live and thrive on the carnivore diet.

This book will teach all you need to know about the carnivore diet, what it entails and why you may want to follow this diet. You will also learn how to begin this diet, why it is a stress-free diet and what benefits you will gain.

Some of the biggest health benefits that seem to come from eating meat only are fat loss, increased metabolism, significantly increased feelings of wellness and energy. Why this occurs has a lot to do with how the body processes WHOLE meat (not processed meat or junk chemically altered meat). We are going to explore how you can start experimenting with this "diet' if you are at an end-roads with your current plan that is not working for you (Fat loss, low energy, losing sub-cutaneous fat, etc..)

Chapter One

What is the Carnivore Diet?

There are plenty of diets and nutrition trends instructing us on the best way to eat. One of the latest is the carnivore diet. This is a pretty simple diet with a simple equation. The equation largely summarizes the diet.

Meat + Water = Carnivore Diet

Introduction to the Carnivore Diet

The carnivore diet is a diet that requires the consumption of only animal food and avoiding everything else.

This diet protocol calls for restricting your carbohydrate intake and eliminate plat food intake completely. It is the direct opposite of a vegan diet but closely resembles the keto diet. Both the carnivore and keto diets rely heavily on proteins and fats as the main source of energy.

The carnivore diet allows you to eat meat and products derived from animals. For instance, you can have fish, beef, meats, eggs, and products such as cream and butter and al other dairy products. However, the diet protocol requires you to avoid other food types like grains, vegetables, nuts, fruits, and seeds.

Complete opposite of a vegan diet

The carnivore diet is a complete opposite of the vegan diet. Science has, for decades, steered us towards pursuit of plant based diets for optimum health and well being while discouraging us from heavy consumption of meats. However, there have been plenty of positive attributes from people following this diet. There are reports from numerous individuals about the health benefits of eating as required by this protocol.

The positive feedback from numerous reports of individuals who've tried this diet has prompted even more people to try it out. The results have been impressive so fat. Some of the positive attributes from people who've tried this diet include faster weight loss, mental clarity, healthier digestive system and improved athletic performance.

The carnivore diet has a simple approach that makes it attractive to anyone searching for a diet that does not come with any complicated nutrition tactics like calculating calories and macros, timing your meals, and so on. The simplicity of this diet and the good reports coming in have made this diet attractive thus far. All that you need to do is to as per this diet is to eat animal foods including beef, fish, eggs, and dairy. You should also stay away from all other foods.

Foods you Should Avoid

Carbohydrates: You need to ensure that you do not take any carbohydrates. These are apparently restricted from the carnivore diet.

Vegetables: You are not supposed to take have vegetables with your diet.

Supplements: you should not take any dietary supplements. The reason for this is that the carnivore diet contains all the minerals and nutrients that the body requires in order to thrive.

Foods you should Eat

Dairy: Dairy is a product derived from animals. It includes diet items like cheese, butter, and milk. You will find, however, that most carnivore dieters prefer to skip dairy or limit its intake due to lactose intolerance that develops in the course of the diet.

Fish: All types of fish are allowed but especially those with lots of fat content. These include fish species like salmon, haddock, and halibut. Seafood is also generally acceptable.

Animal fat products: You can include animal fat products with your diet. These products include tallow, lard, and others so as to enhance your calorie intake.

Meat: You are generally allowed to consume all types of meats. These include red meat, fatty cuts, beef, steak, and all others. These are basically the staples of the carnivore diet. Since carbohydrates are not part of your diet, then you should ensure that you receive the bulk of your nutrition intake from meats.

Meat products

- o Steaks – sirloin, chuck eye, ribeye, strip
- o Ground beef
- o Animal internal organs (optional)
- o Roast – chick, prime rib, brisket

Organ meats: There are some carnivore dieters who are of the opinion that organ meats are essential. The reasoning here is that evidence exists that shows organs aid in the development of human brain. However, not every carnivore dieter is of this opinion. Many prefer taking fish oils, especially oils from cold water fishes like cod. Ideally, you should consider adding cold water fish, liver, and brains to your diet. All these are rich in DHA which is an essential fatty acid. DHA has a vital role in proper functioning of the brain.

Additional Meats

- Lamb – lamb chops, shank, ribs
- Pork – shoulder, pork belly, butt roasts, ribs
- Poultry – wings, drumsticks, thighs, chicken breasts
- Fish – trout, crab, sardines, mackerel, scallops, shrimp, lobster

Beverages

- Bone broth
- Water – with minerals and carbonation or without
- Tea
- Coffee

Coffee is generally regarded as a plant extract. Some carnivore dieters opt to do without it while others freely have it. If you are generally a coffee drinker, then you are free to keep on taking it. Some strict adherents of this diet urge gradual withdrawal. When it comes to meats, you should focus more on grass feed meat and avoid the processed kind. The latter contains additives and preservatives that you do not want in your diet.

How much should you eat?

Basically, you are required to eat as much food as you can. You should eat until you are completely full and whenever you feel hungry. The mantra is to listen to your body and follow what it says.

- o Listen to your body
- o Eat at least two meals per day, more if possible
- o Let your appetite guide you

Even as your body heals and adapts, after years, possibly decades, of malnutrition, you can expect to start eating twice as much as before once your body heals completely. The general guide is to have between two and four ounces of fatty meat each day. Try not to restrict your calorie or food intake and force fasting. This is not part of the carnivore diet and is discouraged.

How do carnivore dieters eat?

A majority of dieters, up to 70%, eat two meals per day. About 10% eat three meals each day while only 20% have 1 meal per day. Ideally, though, you should not count the number of meals that you have in a day. Instead, you should focus on eating whenever you feel hungry and eat until you are full.

Snacks: If you eat sufficient meats throughout the day, then you will probably not see the need to snack during the day. Should you feel hungry then you should increase your meals and eat more during each meal.

Some people tend to snack and do so even when they do not feel hungry. If you really have to snack, then think about pork rinds. Make sure that any meats you eat are not cooked in vegetable fat. In due course, you will realize that most snacking will go away.

A Very Simple Diet

The carnivore diet is one of the simplest diets out there. It encourages you to consume meat only. You do not need to count calories or time your meals. All you need to focus on is eating whenever you feel hungry and eat as much meat as you want. Here is a look at a simple carnivore meal plan.

Breakfast: Bacon with scrambled eggs and tea or black coffee

Lunch: Lamb chops or a t-bone steak

Supper: Porterhouse or 80/20 grass-fed beef

Carnivore Basic Food List

- Unprocessed meat: steak, red meat, fatty meat products
- Fish: especially the oily and fatty kinds like sardines and salmon
- Whole eggs
- Bone marrow
- Bone broth
- Fatty meat products
- Dairy
- condiments

The ideologies of the carnivore diet are based largely on those of the ketogenic diet. There are studies showing that people who eat carbs daily are 30% likely too die compared to those who do not. The same studies showed that those who consume a high fat diet have a 23% less chance of dying compared to those who consume less fat. The study was conducted by researchers at McMaster University.

It is credible studies like these coupled with positive outcomes from dieters that are convincing more and more people to take up the carnivore dieting lifestyle. Take Dr, Anthony Gustin, for instance who is the Perfect Keto Diet founder. Dr.

Gustin's current diet consists of 90% carnivore. He carried out a 30-day experiment and realized his body could stay in ketosis even as he ate meats only.

Chapter Two

The History of the Carnivore Diet

We have been taught ever since we were young that regular meat consumption is fattening, unhealthy, heart-attack inducing, artery clogging, tumor producing, and cholesterol raising and constipating food that should be avoided as much as possible. We were made to believe that a diet full of vegetables and generally plant-based is the most ideal diet on the planet for optimum health.

There is no time in history where human population was confined to a plant-based diet. Neither is there a civilization that depended entirely on a vegan diet. However, there are numerous examples in history of communities that have existed largely on meat-based diets for generations and generations. These families that largely ate meat were never sickly or unhealthy compared to the general populations.

The communities of real people having mostly meat diet for extended periods of time provide us with a lot of insights and powerful information into this diet. We get to learn more about meats and their implications on our bodies and health compared to traditional scientific studies. Conventional scientific studies focus on a small group of individuals for a limited period of time.

Carnivorous Ancestors

If we take a closer look at the diets of our ancestors, we find that there are numerous examples of communities and populations across varied geographical regions and ethnic backgrounds that have opted for a carnivore diet across multiple generations. Here is a look at some examples of communities that practiced a largely carnivorous diet throughout history.

- Maasai from East Africa who consume mainly milk and meat
- Nomads living in Mongolia who lived largely on dairy and meat
- The Sioux of South Dakota ate mostly buffalo meat
- Canadian Inuits whose diet consists largely of fish, whale, seal and walrus
- Gaucho Brazilians who eat mostly meat and beef products
- Russian arctic Chukotka who existed on caribou, fish, and marine animals

Not only did these communities survive on largely meat diets, they thrived. Most of them displayed exceptional strength and health. For instance, the Eskimos from Point Hope ate mostly meat diet consisting of sea cultures, whale, and walrus. According to research, their diet consisted of 35% protein and 50% animal fat.

The researchers discovered that the Point Hope Eskimos had ten times less incidences of heart disease compared to the general population across America. Also, their levels of bad cholesterol were much lower compared to their Caucasian counterparts across continental America.

The Eskimos

Think about the Eskimos, for instance. They had no chance of eating fruit or vegetable any time of the year. Animals such as seals contain zero fiber. By all means, these Eskimo communities ate virtually no vegetables nor fruits. They never tilled the land not harvested crops. Yet they are much healthier than your average person.

While their diets are low in fiber, they are high in animal fat and protein. Such diets generally scare the average American and even institutions like the American Cancer Society, Harvard School of Public Health, and the USDA. Most of these institutions oppose carnivore diets and the consumption of high fat and high protein diets.

A lot of people are puzzled as to how these carnivorous populations obtained their minerals and vitamins without eating any fruits or colorful vegetables. Many wonder how come these communities do not suffer from heart conditions, diabetes, gout, cancers, and other chronic conditions.

To be able to understand how the carnivore diet works, it is advisable to examine closely two different groups of people whose information is readily available. By studying these two groups, it is possible to make some crucial yet fascinating findings relating to the carnivore versus regular diets.

Arctic Communities vs. East African Herdsmen

The Arctic communities live mostly in Alaska, Greenland, Russia, and Canada. The diets of these communities started to change some time in the early 1900s when trade routes and travelers begun introducing foods such as flour, dairy products and flour. These foods did not exist prior to these new trade routes.

In East Africa, we have herdsmen like the Maasai, Samburu, and Pokot. They live around the equator where the temperatures are quite high. According to traditions, the males in these communities lived on only animal products, mostly dairy products and meat. This they do for a period of at least 14 years when the boys turn 28 and become warriors. Teams of American researchers descended into these communities to try and figure out why they were in such exceptional health despite their "unhealthy" diets.

Point Hope in Alaska is a pretty remote location where residents consume a mostly carnivorous diet due to its isolated status. This region was also the subject of a close study by scientists from America. According to the research findings, communities living at this remote location, their diet consisted mostly of walrus and whale meat. An average adult consumed about 3,000 calories per day. Of these 3,000 calories, about 35% was obtained from protein sources while at least 50% was from fat. Carbohydrate intake was limited to about 15 – 20%. This was largely in the form of animal starch or glycogen. The only sugar they had was a type of sucrose sugar that was primarily used to sweeten coffee or tea.

Arctic Findings

Studies were conducted more recently on southwestern Alaskan natives who consumed less traditional foods and more vegetables than their remote counterparts. However, according to the findings of the study, the Alaskans pursuing a traditional diet with more fat and proteins had lower triglyceride levels compared to their southwestern counterparts whose diet consists largely of vegetables and grains with less meat and fat.

Even as recently as the 1980s, very few deaths among the Greenland Eskimos is attributed to heart conditions yet the majority of residents live beyond 60 years of age. There are reports of arctic residents with artery-cholesterol buildup. However, these residents are identified as those who consume a combination of both traditional and modern diets. The high life expectancy of the Eskimos and residents of the arctic is attributed largely to the absence of heart conditions and low cholesterol levels.

Africa Findings

Findings among the African tribes existing largely on a carnivore diet indicate that heart diseases are completely unheard of. Research scientists examined over 600 subjects who were Maasai males. Most of them were 40 years and above. According to this study, only one participant had ever experienced a heart attack. The researchers then examined the hearts of 50 dead Maasai men and found that none of them had passed away due to coronary diseases. Just as with the Eskimos, there was the presence of some cholesterol and fat deposits in some blood vessels but none were serious enough to raise the alarm or cause a blockage.

Among the African communities existing on a carnivore diet, most of the men acquired over 66% of their daily calorie intake from eating animal fat. They consumed about 600 mg of cholesterol and 300 grams of fat each day. Nutritionists and dieticians advise us today to keep our fat intake to between 25 – 35% of our calorie intake and keep out cholesterol amounts to 300 mg per day or less. This means that the African communities were consuming more than twice the recommended amounts without suffering any health consequences.

Effect of Meat on Blood Pressure

Residents of Greenland often consumed a diet rich in animal fat, fish, and meats with very few fruits, dairy products, or vegetables. Sometime in the 1980s and 1990s, some of these people migrated to Denmark and consumed diets high in grains, vegetables, fruits, and other plant products. After a while, researchers discovered that the migrants, now consuming a normal diet, had blood pressure that was 10 points higher than their counterparts back in Greenland.

This was puzzling because they drank less, smoked less, and even weighed a lot less compared to their Greenland counterparts. The crucial point that you need to note here is that consuming less meat while eating more vegetables and fruits, as we are always advised to do, does not necessarily protect or improve health, especially when it comes to blood pressure.

Blood pressure among the East African Maasai

Among the east African nomadic tribes of the Maasai and others, it was discovered by researchers that males aged 15 to 55 averaged a blood pressure of 120/80. It is only about 1% of males who had any significant blood pressure levels that would be of concern. The average weight of the nomadic males was 134 while the average height was 5 foot 7 inches.

The Great Puzzle

It is worth noting then, that communities living off eating meat with plenty of cholesterol and saturated fats are healthy with no weight, blood pressure, or heart problems. Apparently, saturated fats, meats, and cholesterol should be major causes of numerous chronic conditions. On the other hand, vegetables, fruits, and grains protect us from heart conditions and high blood pressure.

So the question is why do communities consuming so much meat, saturated fats and oils fair much better than those consuming supposedly healthier diets consisting of vegetables, fruits, grains, and nuts? While there are no concrete or scientific answers to this and other pertinent questions, it is crucial to note the discrepancy and think about it.

How the Carnivore Diet Works

Animal products like meats are naturally zero carb. This means they do not contain any carbohydrates. When carbohydrate is restricted in our diets, then we lose the need for some nutrients. Also, the vitamins necessary for carbohydrate metabolism become redundant.

A good example is vitamin A. according to a study that focused on this vitamin, it was discovered that in the absence of carbohydrates in the diet, this vitamin was no longer necessary for metabolism regulation. Basically, when we eliminate carbs from the diet, the body will find an alternative source of energy. When this happens, it will enter a phase known as ketosis. In this instance, fat within the body will be converted for energy use. It is thought the body would much rather source its energy from fats via ketosis than any other source. In fact, there are several benefits to the body when ketosis becomes the main source of energy. The carnivore diet operates in an almost similar manner to the keto diet.

However, there are some notable differences. Let us examine some of these differences closely.

Difference between Carnivore Diet and Keto Diet

There are some stark similarities between the keto and carnivore diets. For instance, they both allow regular consumption of proteins and fats while eliminating carbohydrates.

However, the carnivore diet is considered to be a lot more restrictive and takes matters a step further compared to the ketogenic diet. For instance, the keto diet allows you to consume a fair amount of non-animal fatty foods like avocados, coconut oil, and nuts as well as large quantities of plant foods like vegetables.

The ketogenic diet focuses more on high fat and moderate protein intake in order to enable the body enter the ketosis state and start using ketones as the main source of energy for the body. However, the carnivore diet prohibits the intake of other types of fats except animal fat.

Also, the carnivore diet has no macronutrient requirements compared to diets such as keto. However, through this diet, you will still be able to reach ketosis which will be the body's main source of energy.

The keto diet requires you to take 5 – 10% carbohydrates, 20 – 30% proteins, and 60 – 70% fat. In comparison, the carnivore diet has got no such requirements. You do not need to measure or count calories. All you are required to do is eat as much meat as you can until you are full. You are also required to eat whenever you feel hungry but are not restricted to eating only during specified meal times.

There are some dairy foods that are not allowed as part of the ketogenic diet mainly due to higher carbs content. However, in the carnivore diet, all dairy products are permitted because they are derived from animals. The carnivore diet allows all dairy and meat products from animals. These are the main differences between the keto diet and the carnivore diet. However, there are also plenty of similarities.

Adapting to the carnivore diet

The body requires some time before it can adapt to the carnivore diet. Keep in mind that different people have different metabolic rates. Our bodies need to adjust from getting their energy from one source to another. With most people, it takes between two and three weeks for the change to be effective. This is also the same time it takes the average person to start enjoying the benefits of this eating pattern. Those, such as athletes, who have primarily been used to carbs as the main source of energy end up taking much longer to adjust, like three weeks.

Reasons Why Vegetables, Grains, and Fruits are not Allowed

Meat is not necessarily easier to digest but is more nutrient-dense and compact compared to plant matter. Herbivore diet is much more efficient at extracting nutrients. However, such a diet requires that you eat and keep on eating a lot of the time. This is seen in a lot of herbivores. Herbivores have very long digestive systems. A meat only diet does not require you to eat so much throughout the day.

Most vegetables contain toxic enzymes that kill most of the nutrients. This is a self-defense mechanism that most vegetables possess. As a result, you will not get as much nutrients from vegetables because of this. On the other hand, nutrition from meat sources is readily available. You will therefore receive more nutrition from a carnivore diet compared to a herbivore diet consisting of vegetables, grains, and fruits.

Chapter Three

Getting Started with the Carnivore Diet

According to research findings, the carnivore diet is really worth your while. It may sound a little different from what you are used but it actually works. There is plenty of anecdotal testimony out there that supports this way of eating. This is probably why there is a growing shift by conscious individuals including health dieters, athletes, and numerous others towards this way of life.

The main reason why people make the shift to the carnivore diet is because of its numerous benefits. Among these benefits, significant weight loss, an increase in focus and improved moods rank very high with dieters. These are the reasons why this diet is very popular across America and beyond. The carnivore diet also has numerous principles that are very similar to those of a high fat, low carb keto diet. This is also another reason why it is compelling to others. Basically, a diet that restricts your carbohydrate intake is one that is great for you.

Essential Preparation

Before you get started with the carnivore diet, you need to prepare yourself psychologically and physically. A lot of people experiment with this diet for various reasons so it is crucial that you determine why you wish to pursue this eating lifestyle. Let us examine some of the reasons why people choose this diet over all others.

1. Mood: conditions such as depression, focus, bipolar, brain fog and so on

2. Gastro-Intestinal: digestive conditions such as gas, bloating, colitis, heartburn, and gastric reflux

3. Autoimmune disease: conditions like migraines, arthritis, asthma, Lyme's disease, multiple sclerosis and numerous others

4. Keto benefits: benefits like muscle gain, weight loss, and many more

5. Skin conditions: helps with conditions such as acne, rosacea, eczema, psoriasis

Questions

Most people often have questions and doubts about this diet. This is normal and is to be expected. Some of the questions people ask are indicated below.

- How come people on the carnivore diet do not suffer scurvy?
- Can you have proper bowel movements with no fiber?
- What about all the cholesterol?
- Won't this diet surely lead to chronic coronary conditions?
- I will probably end up with cancer, right?

The Adaptation Period

Different people transition differently into the carnivore or all-meat diet. If you were on a keto diet or the HFLC (high fat low carb) diet, then you transition will be easy because your body is probably in keto.

However, if you are transitioning from the standard American diet or SAD which is high in carbohydrates, then it becomes quite difficult to adapt. You should expect some mild challenges during this transition period.

The discomfort that you will experience during the transition period is simply your body's reaction to carbohydrate withdrawal as well as elimination of certain additives, coloring, and chemicals found in processed foods.

Symptoms during Transition

- o Metallic or bad taste in mouth
- o Headaches, brain fog, dizziness
- o Bad breath, bad smells, irritability
- o Digestive issues, sore throat, chills
- o Diarrhea, nausea, soreness, sugar cravings
- o Muscle aches, poor performance, low energy
- o Night sweats, insomnia, rapid heart rate
- o Nocturia or frequent urination at night

What causes all these symptoms?

You may wonder what is going on with your body during the transition period. One of these is something known as fluid rebalancing. The first thing that happens when you cut out carbs is that your insulin levels fall drastically. Once these levels are significantly low, a signal is sent to the kidneys requesting the release of sodium from the body.

You will probably lose about 10 pounds of water in just a couple of days because the water will follow the sodium. The remaining glycogen in your body will eventually be converted into glucose before the body eventually switches to using fatty acids.

From sugar to fat for energy

The body will then begin the transition process from burning mostly glucose for energy to fat. This process needs the body to make a lot of adjustments. Most of these will rely on your metabolic flexibility. This term refers to your body's ability to handle varied sources of energy. People who are accustomed to consuming most carbohydrates will experience feelings similar to withdrawal symptoms like drug addicts do, for instance.

Hormone rebalancing

You are also likely to experience hormonal rebalance and response to the changes take place especially with your metabolism. One of the most significant hormones affected is the T3 thyroid hormone. This hormone is responsible for metabolism, regulation of body temperature, and heart rate. It is also very closely aligned to carbohydrates.

Cortisol plays an important role in the body. For instance, it helps in managing inflammation and is involved in regulating blood sugar levels. Cortisol will be released into the bloodstream as you begin the transition process especially when you start craving sugars and carbs.

During this entire process, the body is actually getting rid of addictions to all the unhealthy carbs and sugars. As the addictions disappear, there will be other changes in your body as well. For instance, you are likely to experience changes in the way the brain transmits signals to your stomach.

This communication channel between your gut and the brain greatly influences a lot of other aspects including neurotransmitters like serotonin and dopamine as well as hormones. These tend to have a huge impact on matters like addictions, cravings, and moods. Going through symptoms akin to withdrawal is not uncommon so you can expect this to happen to you.

Commitment

When you decide you are going to follow this lifestyle, then you should be prepared to make a commitment otherwise it will not work out. Basically, if you are unable to fully commit yourself, then you should wait until such a time as when you will eventually be ready. This may probably be in the form of a condition or possibly a burning desire. Some people on the other hand tend to give up at the slightest sign of discomfort. You should expect a transition period of two weeks or less when your body makes the necessary adjustment.

Prepare for the Transition Period

If you get organized, then you will be able to minimize and even eliminate this transition stage and its numerous symptoms.
You should be prepared

It is crucial that you prepare yourself for this process. Being mentally prepared is definitely advisable so accept and understand the symptoms that you expect to encounter. Once you are mentally prepared, you can also then get physically prepared.

Start eating lots of meat

One of the reasons why you may suffer the symptoms mentioned above is under-eating. Plenty of people do not eat enough because they related this eating lifestyle to other dietary lifestyles that limit food intake. Remember to eat as much meat as you can without restricting intake or tracking macronutrients.

Hydrate throughout the day

The carnivore diet needs you to drink plenty of water throughout the day. As a rule, you need to drink water equivalent to half your bodyweight in ounces. For instance, if you weight 120 pounds, then you need to drink 60 ounces of water each day. Do this especially during the adaption stage. Once the adaption stage is over and you have settled down into this eating style, you should only drink whenever you feel thirsty. Basically you will only drink water when you want to.

Supplement your electrolytes

Another step that you need to follow is to supplement your electrolytes. As your body loses water, you also lose plenty of electrolytes. These include chloride, magnesium, potassium, and sodium. Supplementing is therefore a step that you should take. If you need to supplement, then think about the Pink Himalayan rock salt. It is an excellent source of chloride and sodium. In most cases this should be enough. However, you can also supplement with magnesium and potassium.

You can take supplements that are popular with meat-only dieters. One of these is Ionic Potassium. Alternatively, you can drink meaty bone broth on a regular basis. Bone broth will provide you with lots of the minerals you need including sodium and potassium.

Expect some problem bowel movement

You can expect to encounter gastro-intestinal problems. Apparently these are quite common and mostly for those originally on a low fat diet. Your gall bladder might experience some challenges making the transition. One solution to this problem is choosing lean cuts of meat with very little fat. This is however not a really great idea for a carnivore dieter so follow the solution only for the short term.

Since you are likely to experience bowel movement challenges, you should supplement your diet in this regard. Take a lipase supplement a couple of minutes before your meals. It will help ease your bowel movement challenges and improve your bathroom experience.

If you are coming from a low fat diet, then you might need to take ox bile with your meals in order to ease bowel movement. Sometimes low stomach acid levels can cause problems and you could suffer GERD. Find a supplement to help ease the gastric reflux such as Betaine HCL. This one works really great where others may not be so effective.

Alternatively, you may also consider removing rendered fat from your meats once cooked. Rendered fat is the liquid fat that is produced during cooking. If you notice, in due course of time, that your bowel movements are not as regular or as frequent as they used to be, then just know that this is normal and you are not necessarily constipated. The volume ejected during bowel movement will decrease as the body absorbs meats efficiently with very little waste.

Summary

You need to keep in mind that digestion issues are real and can occur. When they do, you should be prepared to know the right steps to follow. You should supplement your diet as well. Some of the recommended supplements include Betain HCL with Pepsin, ox bile and Lipase. Also remove any rendered fats or at least limit them in your meals.

Prepare for Social Situations

You should prepare yourself for any eventuality but especially for social situations. It is easy to say anything to people you interact with on a regular basis. For instance, you can go on and on about how you eat junk foods and unhealthy meals all day long and they will probably be fine with it.

But the moment you mention that your meals contain no vegetable, no fruit, and essentially no plant-based fruit, they will think you've gone crazy. This is because most people are accustomed to believing that plant-based are essential or else you will suffer serious consequences. Just remember that you owe nobody an explanation about your choices and you should stress about justifying your actions.

However, you can explain that you are trying out a new diet and testing for allergies and things like that. You can say that it is an experiment that you decided to take on just to see how you will fair. Most people are okay with the experiment aspect and will not pursue it further.

Dining out

Dining out is pretty easy because just about all restaurants and eateries have meat on their menus save for vegan ones. You can ask for a burger or steak patty without anything else. Most restaurants and eateries are very understanding, accommodating with fairly-priced meals.

Obtain Sufficient Sleep

Make sure that you get sufficient amounts of sleep each night. You need to get between seven and nine hours of sleep most nights. If you get good sleep regularly, then all other things in your life will get better. At the onset of the carnivore diet, you are likely to experience some level of insomnia. However, this is a phase that will eventually pass. You should learn a couple of hacks that will enable you to sleep better. Here is a look at some of these hacks.

Work out regularly

Exercising is not only therapeutic but also detoxifies your body. It helps the body to expel toxins. Therefore, if you are receiving wonderful nutrition from all the great food you eat, you should give the body a chance to expel toxins. Sweating expels toxins so make sure that you remain fit and active as you follow the carnivore diet. Regular physical activity is a major part of this lifestyle.

Snacking

You should generally not feel the need to take snacks regularly if you eat enough fatty meat at meal times. The rule is, if you continually feel hungry, then you should eat more meat and also eat fattier cuts. A lot of people have made snacking a habit and may not want to stop immediately. People actually snack even when they are not hungry.

If you really must have a snack, then have pork rinds and similar meats. Make sure that they are not fried or prepared in vegetable oil. According to experience, though, snacking tends to disappear over time. So you can expect your need to have a regular snack fade eventually.

The Carnivore Cleanse

The carnivore cleanse is a revolutionary new way of living where you cleanse your systems, detoxify the body and heal through diet. It is a natural way of eating that supports detoxification and body cleansing.

You will allow the body a much-needed break from all processed, unnatural foods, junk food, as well as grains and carbs. Your body will heal immensely and after a period of time, your health will improve. You will become healthier and will feel like a million dollars.

Chapter Four

The Three Levels of the Carnivore Diet

The carnivore diet is actually a very simple diet. In fact, it is too simple with an equally simple equation that sums it up perfectly.

Carnivore Diet = Meat + Water

Yet this simple equation evokes a lot of questions. There are lots of people wondering whether this diet is sufficient for all their nutrition needs. Ideally, you should start very slowly and progress steadily with time your body learns to tolerate this diet.

Remember to eat as often as possible and to eat till full. However, it will be totally up to you to decide whether to have three, two, or a single meal per day.

The Different Levels of Carnivore Diet

The carnivore diet is best viewed at three different levels. These levels do not aim to make this diet a complex one but simply provide you with a framework that makes it easier for you regardless of your situation. These different levels are level 1, level 2, and level 3.

Level 2 and level 3 are ideally designed to assist you to find the intolerances and sensitive issues that are present due to a diet that causes chronic inflammation. These two levels help you to purify the diet in a way that enables you to then add other foods. These are foods that probably give you more energy, a clear head, excellent health and so on.

As an example, you could be allergic to pork but totally unaware of it. However, this fact could be discovered and eliminated at levels 2 or 3. A lot of dieters thrive at the first level or level 1. It is advisable that you take a few weeks at each level to enable you to determine which foods suit you best and what diseases or adverse symptoms persist.

Level 1 Protocol

At level 1, your diet should consist generally of meat. Anything that is meat or fish or a product of either qualifies to be at this level. There are some exceptions here and these include tea and coffee as well as eggs, butter, whipping cream and cheese.

You can add some dietary supplements at this level. The most suitable supplements during the adaptation stage are electrolytes, pink Himalayan salt, and others such as ox bile, Lipase or Betaine HCL.

You should ensure that you stick with your standard carnivore protocol until you have truly adapted to the diet.

Level 2 Protocol

At level 2, things will be a little bit different. You will have to strictly eat natural meat and meat products only. For instance, you cannot have any processed meats. These are not goo for you because they contain preservatives, additives, and possibly coloring. Avoid processed meats as much as possible.

You should also avoid exceptions and non-meat side snacks. This means you cannot have side dishes like whipping cream, cheese, butter, eggs, coffee or tea. You may also not supplement your diet. At this stage, you are trying to eliminate all these additional foods to observe your body's reaction.

There are some exceptions though because you are allowed to supplement with pink Himalayan salt. You are also allowed some supplements if you are starting at level 2 while skipping level 1.

Level 3 Protocol

At this level, your body will have been used to the diet and will be ready to refine it. This is why you will be expected to consume only grass feed beef and water.
Therefore, expect to feed only on beef and drink only water.

This level is also known as the ultimate carnivore diet and it will help you eliminate all other products, specifically meats that your body may be sensitive to. There are people that are sensitive to pork others are sensitive to certain types of fish and sea foods, and so on. When you consume only high quality beef, then you will easily be able to learn which animals are good for you and which ones are not. You will also be able to track all intolerances you may have and why they occurred.

In brief, at this final level, you should eliminate all other meats and meat products and only have grass fed and grass finished beef. You should also drink water only. Cut out the dairy products, the processed meats, and all others. Eating grass fed meat only is not cheap and will cost you plenty of money. However, it is well worth it.

Beyond the three different levels, you will be in excellent position to perfect and personalize your own diet. You can ideally now begin to look back and see which foods are problematic and which ones are excellent for you. Simply evaluate the foods and how you feel when you eat each. Here is the process;

1. First add regular beef back to your diet (non-grass fed)
2. Next step is to test other meats and see how your body reacts
3. Now try out some eggs and observe your body's reaction
4. Give dairy a try
5. Finally, try both coffee and tea and note your body's reaction

Once you complete the third level for instance, you may choose to add lamb chops or chicken to your diet. When you eventually do, you should also be on the lookout for any symptoms, discomfort and so on.

For instance, let us say you add pork and notice that you feel bloated. In such a case, you should cut it out. Stop eating any product that probably makes you feel any kind of discomfort. If there is any particular meat or meat product that makes you feel great, then you should definitely keep it.

The aim here is to personalize your diet and eating plan to suit your body. Your baseline for the test will be grass fed and finished beef. If you try a eat product and it is okay then you should be free to keep it.

Where to Begin

Ideally, you should start at level 1. This level is the best for all beginners even if you were already on the ketogenic diet. The keto diet is thought to be very close to the carnivore diet.

Sometimes it is advisable for anyone who is not a coffee drinker to begin the carnivore diet at level 2. The reason for this is that it offers the necessary flexibility but without the challenges encountered by those originally on no diet or standard American diet. You should endeavor to spend at least one entire month at a given level before advancing. For instance, if you start at level 1, you should spend at least 30 days at this level before advancing to level 2 and spending a further thirty days here.

Beyond Level 3

Once dieters complete the third level, they usually choose to settle at level one. Majority opt for level 1 while others prefer level 2. Level 1 is less restrictive and accommodates plenty of other products besides grass fed beef. It is crucial that you always remember the baseline for this diet is grass fed as well as finished beef. If you managed to get to level 3 and complete thirty days here, then you will easily be able to determine at which level you belong.

You need to keep in mind that while most people will have settled into the diet after initial metabolic challenges, others may take months to settle down. It is advisable to test for longer just so as to gauge how great the diet is for you and what adjustments you will need to make.

Surviving to the end of level 3 after starting at level one is not an easy feat so congratulations is you manage it. Lots of people sometimes cheat while others are unable to complete all three levels. However, if you know what you want and have your priorities right, then you should be successful eventually.

How to Survive the First Month

The carnivore diet demands that you eat meat and animal products for every meal each day. This amounts to plenty of fat, lots of protein and no carbs. The challenge with this approach is that the body is accustomed to believe grains, fiber, and vegetables are essential nutrients. If this were the case, then conventional wisdom would imply that carnivore dieters experience excessive weight gain, digestive problems, high cholesterol, and other problems.

Fortunately, conventional wisdom is not always accurate. If you closely examine the carnivore diet, you will notice that it is very similar to what our ancestors ate. Many centuries ago, our ancestors ate plenty of meat because it did not make sense to them to gather plenty of vegetables and fruits. Because of this, our bodies became seriously accustomed to a meat-oriented diet.

Historical Observation by Dr. George Ede MD

The world is yet to produce any civilization that ate a vegetarian diet from birth to death. However, there are numerous examples in history of people from varied ethnic, cultural, and geographical backgrounds who ate mostly meat diets for numerous years, lifetimes, and across generations.

Interesting Facts about the Carnivore Diet

Plenty of people love meat and other fatty foods. A diet consisting mostly of meaty foods is easy for most people to consider. Your body goes into ketosis when you eat very little or no carbs at all. Ketosis has been associated with plenty of benefits such as strength gain, weight loss, and mental health challenges like ADHD.

One of the things that you need to avoid is take certain foods even in moderation. For instance, if you eat anything containing sugar or starch, then you may want more. A little sugar is likely to make you desire more. The best solution is to not touch sugar at all. While you may experience some withdrawal symptoms at first, these will subside significantly in due course of time.

On other diets, some cravings might occur and dieters are allowed to cheat occasionally. However, with the carnivore diet, all cravings will very likely disappear and you will not need to have a cheat meal. You will eventually be able to eat your meals without the desire to have other foods, especially junk foods.

Losing weight following the carnivore diet is not just possible but actually comes easy. By religiously pursuing this eating lifestyle, you will drop the pounds and develop strong yet lean muscle.

Challenges and how to overcome them

It is advisable to be aware of the kind of challenges to expect when starting the carnivore diet. Most of these may have been discussed in a different chapter. However, here are a couple of things that you need to be keen on.

You should first go and get your blood tested. You will need to then go back and get tested a second time after about three months. This way, you will be able to note and measure the effects of the diet. You may also want to speak to your doctor or a nutritionist before trying out anything.

Once you begin trying out this diet, you should take note of any changes in your weight, digestive system, and energy levels. Each individual is different and people are affected differently by food and diet. Most people who've tried the carnivore diet have benefited immensely from it. Even then, you should still maintain contact with a healthcare practitioner just so that you stay safe.

Initial week

The first week will most likely also be your toughest. At this stage, you can expect to experience fluctuations in your energy levels, appetite and even focus. To ease this transition, start your journey at a time when you are not too busy but in great overall health. Make sure that you can operate from home, at least for the initial week, or take time off your regular schedule. If you must, ensure that you give yourself sufficient time to sleep.

It is possible to experience certain unexpected challenges. For instance, someone lost appetite for beef yet it is the main ingredient of the carnivore diet. There are numerous reasons that could cause this. However, you should try other options such as lamb chops, chicken, and so on. You can store alternatives like cheese that will help you when you need to snack.

Sometimes the need to cheat during the first week arises. You should try as hard as possible to stay clean and not cheat at all. However, if you really have to cheat, then do so with foods that are not too far from the carnivore diet. For instance, you can have some peanut butter or hazel nuts. While they are not a part of the diet, they are close to it. Compare this to something far out like a rich cream cake.

Appetite swings

You should prepare yourself for occasional appetite swings. On some days you will be able to go several hours without eating. On other days, you may feel hungry just a few hours after a major meal. It is likely though that your appetite will level out after the first couple of weeks so try and hang in there till then. In that time, you will probably have figured out portion sizes for your meals. You should ensure that you have access to quality carnivore food all day everyday.

Some Frequently Asked Questions

Everybody has plenty of questions to ask about this diet especially if they are very new to it. You probably have lots of questions of your own as well. This is common and you should not be afraid to ask questions. Here are some common questions about the carnivore diet.

1. *Are vegetables are allowed with this diet?*

The answer is a distinct no. While you may have all along thought that vegetables are crucial to good health, they may not be that important. Vegetables are a good source of minerals and vitamins but they may not be the best. They tend to contain anti-nutrients which prevent uptake of the nutrients by the body. Veggie nutrients are also largely destroyed by cooking.

2. *How do you manage without fiber?*

According to experts, if you do not eat plenty of junk food and processed foods, then you will probably not need that much fiber. Basically, fiber is helpful but in this instance where your food is natural, it may not be that necessary.

3. *Are you not worried about cholesterol levels?*

There is ongoing debate in academic circles as to whether animal fat and meat cause high cholesterol. Cholesterol is affected by plenty of variables. These tend to have a profound effect on your body. There is a huge difference if you take a lot of fat and sugar compared to eating a high fat diet with no sugar. This means that it is the sugar that is the source of the problem and not the fat.

4. *Isn't red meat harmful to your body?*

There are often plenty of variables at play in life. If you consume plenty of sugary foods and red meat but don't exercise, then your health will definitely be affected. However, if you eat red meat, avoid sugar completely, and workout regularly, then you will be in excellent shape.

5. *Should I expect to experience any digestive problems?*

It is normal to expect digestive problems with any diet that excludes vegetables. With the carnivore diet, you can expect to only encounter minor discomforts which are quit insignificant compared to other diets. And most of these discomforts will disappear on their own and will generally only be a nuisance than a real cause for concern.

6. *Will I need to supplement with micronutrients?*

Supplementing with micronutrients is not really necessary especially for the first couple of weeks and months. The aim during the initial stages is to find out how the diet affects micronutrients especially during the first few weeks. Therefore dietary supplements should really be out of question. If you supplement, then you will never get to learn about the deficiencies, if any, or major benefits of this diet.

7. *Are organ meats allowed?*

Yes, of course. Organ meats should constitute part of your diet. Not only are they highly nutritious but are also very tasty. They provide you with an extra shield of nutrients which your body desperately needs. Organ meats can also be viewed as insurance against any potential nutritional deficiencies.

8. *How about the kidneys and all that protein?*

There is a myth in the world of nutrition that kidneys and proteins do not get along. It is also a part of the misinformation that tends to discourage dieters from partaking of this diet. There is basically no truth that proteins will adversely affect your kidneys.

9. *Is this diet more or less expensive compared to the standard diet?*

Most people think that costs of both diets are more or less the same. The standard American diet may be cheaper in some instances but costs do not vary that much. Even then, high quality meats and fats are quite costly. Grass-fed cattle and wild caught meat is more expensive compared to grain-fed animals.

Chapter Five

Best Meals for the Carnivore Diet

All-meat or carnivore diet is growing in popularity. Plenty of well-known celebrities and non-celebrities alike are pursuing this diet in one form or another. One of them is Mikhaila Peterson who is the daughter of Jordan B. Peterson. She's on a carnivore diet to ward of an autoimmune disease that almost killed her as a child. Here is a look at some great carnivore meals that you can have any time of day or night.

Breakfast Carnivore Meals

1. California grilled chicken

Ingredients

- Freshly ground black pepper
- Kosher salt
- 1 tsp garlic powder
- Italian seasoning
- 4 pieces of skinless, boneless, chicken breasts
- 4 slices of mozzarella cheese

Directions

Take a small bowl and mix together garlic powder with Italian seasoning, oil, salt and pepper. Pour this mixture over the chicken and let it marinate for 20 to 30 minutes.

Pre-heat the grill and add the seasoned and marinated chicken breasts. Grill the pieces until properly charred and cooked through. It should take 8 minutes to properly cook each side. Now pour in the mozzarella cheese and grill for another two minutes.

2. Philly Cheese Steaks

Ingredients

- o   1 lb thinly sliced flank steak
- o   2 cloves of garlic, diced
- o   4 slices of provolone cheese
- o   Kosher salt
- o   Freshly ground black pepper
- o   Freshly chopped parsley
- o   2 tbsp Italian seasoning
- o   2 tbsp animal oil

Directions

Heat the grill to medium heat. Take a large bowl and mix together the garlic, steak, pepper, animal oil, and season with salt and black pepper. Now place the mixture in foil packs.

Fold up the packs nicely and put them in the grill. Grill the steak for about 10 minutes. It should be nicely cooked now. Open the grill and add the cheese. Let the cheese melt into the steak. Allow to cook for a further two minutes. Garnish with parsley and serve.

3. Scrambled Eggs and Milk

Ingredients

- o   A pinch of salt
- o   Freshly ground black pepper
- o   Some animal fat/oil
- o   2 medium-size eggs
- o   1 glass of milk

Preparation

Heat a shallow pan or skillet over medium heat on a stove. Pour in some of the fat and let it heat for a minute. Take the eggs and break over the pan or skillet. Use a wooden or plastic spoon to prevent the egg from sticking onto the pan.

Place the egg onto a plate and season with the salt and pepper. Now warm the milk in a sauce pan and then pour it into a glass.

4. Pork Shoulder Cutlets

Ingredients
- 1.5 pounds of boneless pork shoulder divided into 4 parts
- 2 large eggs
- ¾ cups all-purpose flour
- ¾ cup animal oil
- Sea salt
- Freshly ground pepper

Preparation

Take the pork steaks and pound between double layer plastic wrap. Take a bowl and lightly beat the eggs. Add some cornstarch and season with the freshly ground black pepper as well as the kosher salt.

Take the cutlets and season individually with pepper and kosher salt. Transfer to the egg mixture and coat them generously. Take a skillet and put on the stove at medium heat. Heat some of the oil and cook the cutlets two at a time. Allow them to cook for three minutes at a time. You may now remove them from the heat and place on a wire rack then season with pepper and salt.

6. Pan Ranch Pork Chops

Ingredients

- 4 pieces of 8-ounce pork chops
- 2 tbsp of oil
- Packaged ranch seasoning
- 3 cloves of sliced and diced garlic
- Freshly ground black pepper
- Kosher salt

Directions

First pre-heat the oven till 400 degrees F. Take a baking sheet, oil it lightly and then place the pork chops on it. Pour some more oil and add the salt and pepper to taste. Take the Ranch Seasoning and add to the pork chops.

Place the baking sheet with the seasoned pork chops into the oven. Let them cook for a while until well and thoroughly cooked. They will get to an internal temperature of about 140 degrees F when properly cooked. Now broil for about two to three minutes until the meat turns a nice brown color or becomes slightly charred. The meat is now ready to serve. The cooking time for this particular meal will depend on the thickness or size of the pork chops.

7. Baked Chicken Fingers

Ingredients

- o 1 pound of skinless, boneless chicken cutlets
- o Kosher salt
- o Freshly ground black pepper
- o 2 large, beaten eggs
- o 3 tbsp animal oil

Directions

First pre-heat the oven to a temperature of 425 degrees F then take a baking sheet and line it with foil. Take the chicken cutlets and cut them into strips of about one and a half inches. Season the cutlets with salt and pepper.

Dip the chicken strips in the eggs and then transfer the strips to the baking sheet. Now, once all the chicken strips are on the baking sheet, let them cook in the hot oven for 10 to 12 minutes or until they turn golden brown. Now heat broiler until it turns a nice golden brown.

Your chicken is now ready so remove from the oven, place on a plate carefully and serve whilst still nice and hot. Enjoy the chicken fillets.

8. Fish Fingers

Ingredients

- 2.5 pounds fish fillet
- 1 cup flour
- 2 beaten eggs
- ½ tsp of garlic powder
- Kosher salt
- Freshly ground black pepper

2 tbsp Animal fat

Directions

Take a deep frying pan and pre-heat the oil. Slice the fish into long, thin, strips.
Combine the garlic powder with some salt, flour, and pepper in a bowl. Beat the eggs thoroughly in another bowl.

Now dip the fish fingers in the salt, flour, and pepper mixture. Make sure that they are evenly coated. Put the fish fingers in the pan and fry till golden brown or for about 2 to 3 minutes. Remove from the pan and place on a plate. Serve while hot.

9. Grilled lamb chops

Ingredients

- 2 tbsp garlic powder
- A pinch of cayenne powder
- Sea salt
- 2 tbsp animal fat/oil
- 6 lamb chops about ½-inch thick

Procedure

Use a food processor and add the assorted spices then combine them so they mix properly. Add the animal fat and mix further. Take the paste and apply it onto the lamb chops. Allow them to marinade for about an hour.

Take a grill pan and place it on the stove at high heat. Add the chops and let the sear for 2 to 3 minutes. Now turn them over and sear some more for another 2 to 3 minutes. They should be cooked now so place them on a plate and serve while hot.

10. Teriyaki Chicken Wings

Ingredients

- 12 pieces of chicken wings rinsed and dried
- 2 tbsp animal fat/oil
- 1 tbsp toasted sesame seeds
- Freshly ground black pepper
- Kosher salt
- Teriyaki sauce

Preparation

Pre-heat your oven to a temperature of 400 degrees F.
Take the chicken wings and season them adequately with the salt and pepper. Pour a little oil on them and let them sit for a couple of minutes.

Take a baking sheet and lay the wings. Put the sheet in the oven and bake for about half an hour or until the wings turn a nice brown color and are cooked through.

Prepare your meat only sauce and simmer on low heat. Enjoy the chicken wings with the sauce while still hot.

Carnivore Lunch Meals

1. Grilled Buffalo Wings

Ingredients

- 1 tsp freshly ground black pepper
- 1 tsp of garlic powder
- 3 lbs whole chicken wings
- 1 tsp kosher salt
- 1/3 cup of hot sauce
- 1 tbsp honey
- 6 tbsp butter

Directions

Take a small bowl and combine the pepper, salt and garlic powder. Take a large bowl and put the wings then add the seasoning mixture of salt, garlic, and pepper. Make sure the chicken wings are evenly coated.

Pre-heat a grill oven to a temperature of 350 degrees F. Take the wings and place them in the grill. Make sure that they are closely touching each other. This is the complete opposite of conventional grilling where space between the pieces is necessary to prevent steaming.

In this case, steaming is necessary to keep them moist. Flip the wings occasionally and grill for about 20 minutes. Take a shallow pan and heat the butter, honey, and hot sauce on low heat. Whisk the mixture so the ingredients mix thoroughly.

Take the wings out of the oven toss them in the sauce ensuring they are generously coated and place back in the oven. Allow them to sit in the oven for an additional 2 minutes then serve while hot.

2. Grilled Strip Steaks

Ingredients

- 1 tsp dried garlic powder
- 3 strip steaks 1.5 inches thick
- 1 tsp chipotle Chile powder
- 1.5 tbsp animal fat
- 1 tsp red pepper flakes
- Freshly ground black pepper
- Kosher salt

Directions

Take a small bowl and combine the black pepper with the kosher salt, chipotle powder, garlic and red pepper flakes. Mix the ingredients thoroughly and then let it sit.

Take the steaks and pat them dry using paper towels. Then place the steaks in a mid-sized baking dish. Rub the steaks with some oil and then pour some seasoning generously on them. Make sure that all the pieces are generously covered with the seasoning mix.

Now cover the bowl and let it sit for about an hour or two so that the flavors can penetrate the steaks. Once the steak pieces are properly marinated, heat the grill and place the steaks on a tray. Place the tray in the grill and let the steaks cook for a couple of minutes. Turn each side after two minutes and then turn again so that all sides are cooked.

Once the steaks are nicely cooked, transfer them to a plate and cover them tightly using aluminum foil. Let the steaks rest for a couple of minutes. Now remove the foil after a quarter of an hour. If not then the steaks will continue to cook. Take a large knife and slice the steaks. Check if the salt is sufficient and sprinkle some more if necessary. Serve while hot.

3. Parmesan Chicken Cutlets

Ingredients

- o   2 large eggs
- o   ¼ cup grated Parmesan cheese
- o   1.5 cups Japanese breadcrumbs
- o   4 pieces of boneless, skinless, chicken cutlets
- o   2 tbsp Animal oil
- o   1 tbsp Mustard powder
- o   Freshly ground black pepper
- o   Kosher salt

Preparation

Take a shallow bowl and beat the eggs. Use another bowl and add the parmesan cheese and mustard powder. Season the mixture with both salt and pepper. Take the chicken pieces and season with the kosher salt and black pepper.

Dredge the chicken pieces in flour and shake off the excess. Put the chicken pieces in the bowl with the beaten eggs and ensure they are well coated. Remove from the egg bowl and add to parmesan cheese bowl.

Heat the oil in a large skillet over medium-heat. Cook the cutlets and add some more oil. Let it cook for about 4 minutes. Once cooked, place the chicken pieces on paper towel-lined plate.

4. Monster Meat Balls

Ingredients
- 1 cup of milk
- ½ pounds of ground turkey
- 2 tbsp of garlic powder
- ¼ cup parsley for garnish
- 1 large diced and sliced onion
- Parsley
- 2 cups of grated parmesan cheese
- 2 tbsp animal oil

Preparation

Take the turkey and place it in a bowl. Add some parmesan cheese, garlic, parsley, pepper and some salt. Pour in some milk and mix together. Add some bread crumbs to help bind the ingredients and form meat balls. Now form three or four oversized meatballs.

Turn on the oven and heat some oil on medium heat. Take the meatballs whilst still in the small pot and place them in the oven. Let them sear over the surface for a while and keep moving them around. This helps to maintain their round shape.

Now remove the meatballs from the oven and add the sauce and some water. Ensure that they are covered completely by the sauce and place back in the oven. Let is sit for a while and allow it to simmer. Cover the sauce pan as the turkey meatballs simmers and ensure to keep turning them occasionally.

5. Beef Stew

Ingredients

- 2 tbsp oil
- 2.5 pounds of beef chuck sliced into 2-inch cubes
- Freshly ground black pepper
- Kosher salt
- 2 tbsp garlic powder
- Some flour
- Fresh spices
- 10 cups of beef or chicken broth or water

Directions

Heat the large Dutch oven over medium heat. Generously pour some animal oil in the pan and fill it about ¼ of the way up. Use the salt and pepper to season the beef pieces and then add them to the pan. Now sauté some of the beef pieces and stir occasionally. Keep going until the pieces turn a nice brown color. This will probably take about 8 minutes.

Now sauté the rest of the beef pieces and a further 8 minutes later transfer the beef from the pan to a plate.

6. BBQ Chicken Drumsticks

Ingredients

- 1 teaspoon of paprika
- Freshly ground black pepper
- Kosher salt
- 12 pieces of chicken drumsticks
- 2 tbsp garlic powder
- ½ a cup of water
- Some oil or animal fat

Directions

Take a small bowl and mix together the paprika, salt, black pepper, and any other seasoning. Use this spicy mixture to season the drumsticks. Make sure that you loosen the skin before seasoning the meat. Once you have nicely and generously seasoned all the drumsticks, cover them carefully using plastic wrap then let them marinate overnight or for at least an hour.

Get the grill ready and pre-heat to medium heat. Use the oil on the grill grate to prevent the chicken drums from sticking. Proceed to grill the chicken and keep turning it until it is properly and thoroughly cooked. Check that the skin is crisp. This should take about 25 or so minutes. Remove from the grill once ready and place them on a plate. Serve the drumsticks while still hot.

7. Mexican Fish Stew

Ingredients

- 4 tilapia fish fillets, each cut into 4 pieces
- Freshly ground pepper and kosher salt
- 2 tbsp animal fat/oil
- 2 tbsp ground garlic powder
- 1 tbsp chili powder

Directions

Take a shallow dish and put in the fish fillet pieces. Get the seasoning and season the fish generously. This includes the salt, pepper, and garlic powder. Now take a large skillet and put it on the stove on medium heat. Add some oil and seasoning then put the fish to the skillet.

Get some hot water or broth and add to the fish. Let it cook and stir slightly until cooked. Check for seasoning and add some more salt or pepper if necessary. Your Mexican fish stew is now ready to serve. Serve while hot.

8. Marinated Chicken Breasts

Ingredients

- 3 tsp dried herbs
- 2 tbsp vinegar
- 2 tsp garlic powder
- Freshly ground pepper and kosher salt
- 4 pieces of skinless, boneless chicken breasts
- ¼ cup of oil

Directions

Take the vinegar and assorted herbs and powders and pour them into a sealable plastic bag. Add some oil to the mixture then shake the bag and all its ingredients. Ensure that the ingredients mix thoroughly.

Now open the bag and place the chicken breast pieces inside. Shut the bag and shake it thoroughly so that the oil and seasoning mixture coats the chicken pieces evenly. You can freeze these for a while if you like.

Remove the plastic bag from the freezer, thaw in the microwave, then place on a pan. Heat a grill pan or grill and when it turns hot place the chicken breast pieces. Let the chicken cook for at least 4 minutes then turn sides and cook for a further 4 minutes. Ensure that the pieces are properly cooked. The chicken is now ready to serve.

9. Oven Roasted Lamb Shanks

Ingredients

- 3 tbsp animal oil
- Freshly ground black pepper and kosher salt
- 4 pieces of lamb shanks
- 4 tbsp mixed herbs
- 3 cups of water

Directions

Preheat the oven then heat the animal oil over high heat in a medium Dutch oven until the oil starts to smoke. Take the shanks and pour the mixed herbs seasoning on both sides. Add to the heat and let them sear until they turn into a beautiful golden brown color on both sides.

Once the golden brown beautiful color is observed, the shanks are ready and can be removed and placed onto a plate. Prepare a soup, broth, or sauce and then enjoy the lamb shanks with the broth.

10. Mexican Chicken Soup

Ingredients

- 2 whole or 4 split chicken breasts with skin and bone
- Some animal oil
- 3 tbsp garlic powder
- 2 tbsp mixed dry herbs
- 1 tsp ground cumin
- 1 tsp coriander seed

Instructions

Preheat your oven at a temperature of 350 degrees F. Take a sheet pan then place the chicken breasts on it. Pour some oil then sprinkle some pepper and salt. Roast the chicken breasts for about 40 minutes. Once cooked let it sit for a while then remove the bones and skin.

Shred the meat then cover it and put it aside. Now you can prepare your favorite broth or warm some if you have. Put the broth in a saucepan, place on the stove on medium heat then add the chicken pieces. Season the mixture to taste using the mixed herbs then add some more salt and pepper if necessary.

Let the soup boil and then lower the heat. Let it simmer for about 5 to 7 minutes before removing from the heat. Your chicken soup is now ready to serve. You should serve it hot and enjoy this delicious meal.

Dinner Carnivore Meals

1. Hawaiian Roasted Pork

Ingredients

- 2 tbsp freshly ground black pepper
- 3 tbsp coarse or Hawaiian salt
- 2 pieces of boneless pork rump roasts
- 2 tbsp of oil
- Natural herbs

½ cup of water
10 wet banana leaves
1 tbsp mixed natural herbs

Instructions

Place the pork roasts on a plate and season them with the pepper and salt. Prepare an outdoor barbecue using wood chips soaked in water and add to the coals.

Place the pork on the hot grill and sear in order to lock in all the natural juices. Season the pork with the natural herbs. Take 5 banana leaves and place them on the foil paper then place the roasts on top. Fold the banana leaves and then roast the pork for a further 3 hours and cover the grill. It should now be ready to serve so shred the meat using two forks.

2. Pan Fried Tilapia

Ingredients

- ½ tsp fresh ground black pepper
- 1 teaspoon sea salt
- 1.5 pounds of fresh tilapia fish fillets
- ¼ cup flour
- 2 tsp mixed seasoning
- 2 tbsp butter
- 1 tsp ground garlic

Instructions

Preheat the oven to about 300 degrees F. Take a shallow baking dish and thoroughly mix the seasoning with pepper, salt, flour, and salt. Place the tilapia fillets in the seasoning and coat both sides generously. Shake off any excess then place the fish in a skillet.

Sear the fish on both sides for about 2 minutes each side. Once both sides turn a nice brown color, remove from the skillet and transfer to a baking sheet lined with paper towels or a paper grocery bag. Put the fish in the oven to maintain the warmth.

Turn down the heat to low and then add the butter. Let the butter melt all over the fish in order to add flavor. Add more of the natural herbs and allow to sauté for about 2 minutes. Remove the fish and place on a platter or serving plates.

3. Grilled Prime Ribs

Ingredients

- o 2 tbsp garlic powder
- o Freshly ground black pepper
- o 3 prime rib-eye steaks
- o Mixture of dried seasoning
- o Some animal based cooking oil

Instructions

Preheat the grill to 350 degrees F. Take the steaks and season them generously in a bowl. Ensure that both sides are seasoned with the salt, pepper, and the seasoning. After the seasoning, set aside and let it sit.

Form a paste using the garlic and set it aside. Now take a small skillet and place it on the stove over medium heat and add some oil. Once the oil starts heating up, add the garlic paste and stir thoroughly. Now allow the oil to come to a boil then let it simmer for a while. Add some seasoning and then cook until it turns a nice golden brown color.

Remove the skillet from the heat and let the garlic cool still in the oil. Mix it some more till it becomes a paste. Now put the meat on top of a hot grill then cook till it turns a nice brown color on both sides. It should take about 5 minutes for one side and 3 minutes for the other side.

Take the garlic paste and smear over the meat. Make sure that the steaks are facing upwards and place on the grill rack in the stove. Cook some more for about 10 minutes for rare. Remove from the grill and let it sit for about 10 minutes. Transfer the meat from the grill onto a chopping board then proceed to cut the meat between the bone and flesh of each steak. It is now ready to serve.

4. Perfect Roast Turkey

Ingredients

- 1 tbsp assorted dry spices
- ¼ lbs of unsalted butter
- 1 large, fresh turkey weighing 15 – 20 lbs
- Freshly ground pepper and kosher salt
- 2 tbsp Dried garlic and onion

Procedure

First pre-heat the oven to a temperature of 350 degrees F. Now melt the butter in a small pan and add the seasoning. Set this mixture aside. Take the turkey and wash it thoroughly after removing the giblets. Remove any leftover feathers if present then dry the outside by patting.

Take a large roasting pan and place the turkey in it. Pour some salt and pepper on the inside of the turkey cavity. Now pour some seasoning on the inside as well. Take the butter mixture and brush the turkey on the outside. Now tie the turkey legs together using tuck and string beneath the bird.

Roast the turkey in the grill for about 3 hours or until the juices run clear if you cut the turkey between the thigh and the leg. Take the turkey from the grill and place it on a cutting board. Ensure that you cover it with aluminum foil to maintain the heat and juices. Let the bird rest for about 20 to 30 minutes. Find some large sharp knives then slice the turkey the right way. It is now ready to serve.

5. Goat meat Stew

Ingredients

- 2 tbsp oil
- 2.5 pounds of goat meat chuck sliced into 2-inch cubes
- Freshly ground black pepper
- Coarse kosher salt
- 2 tbsp garlic powder
- Fresh spices
- 10 cups of goat or chicken broth or water

Directions

Heat a large Dutch oven over medium heat. Generously pour some animal fat or oil in the pan and fill it about ¼ of the way up. Use the salt and pepper to season the beef pieces and then add them to the pan.

Now sauté some of the goat meat pieces and stir occasionally. Keep going until the pieces turn a nice brown color. This will probably take about 8 minutes. Now sauté the rest of the meat pieces and a further 8 minutes later transfer the beef from the pan to a plate.

6. Pan-fried Beef Liver

Ingredients

- o   1 tbsp ground garlic
- o   2 tbsp freshly ground black pepper
- o   2 tbsp coarse sea salt
- o   1 large beef liver, cut up into small cubic chunks
- o   1 cup dried mixed herbs
- o   ¼ cup animal oil

Procedure

Place the beef liver pieces in a bowl. Add salt and pepper then pour in the seasoning. Mix it thoroughly then set it aside for about 15 minutes. Take a skillet and put it on the stove at medium heat. Add the oil and heat if for about a minute.

Now pour in the liver and all the seasoning. Reduce the heat to low and let it cook for about 10 minutes. Cover the skillet so as to hold in the flavors. Check it occasionally and add some water. Pour in the garlic powder then cover and leave for 2 to 3 more minutes.

Take the skillet off the heat and set it aside. The liver should be cooked and should have a nice, thick stew. Taste and add some salt or pepper if necessary. Your beef liver is now ready to serve.

7. Bacon and Cheese Omelet

Ingredients

- Freshly ground black pepper
- ¼ cup parmesan cheese
- 1 tsp ground garlic
- 2 large eggs
- Coarse sea salt
- 3 slices of bacon
- 1 tbsp animal oil

Instructions

Cut up the bacon into thin strips. Season the bacon strips and set aside. Chop up the parmesan cheese. Set aside as well. Take a pan and put it on the stove on low heat. Pour some oil on the pan.

Take a small bowl and beat the eggs. Add salt and pepper to taste. Pour the beaten eggs onto the pan and spread out. Add the bacon onto the eggs and let it cook for just a couple of seconds. Now pour in the parmesan cheese together with the dried garlic.

Turn the omelet and allow the other side to cook. This should cook for about 1 minute and the omelet is ready. The bacon strips should turn a nice brown color. Check for salt and sprinkle some more if necessary. Place the omelet on a plate and you are now ready to serve.

8. Grilled Tuna Steaks

Ingredients

- 2 tbsp fish or animal oil
- Freshly ground black pepper
- Coarse sea salt
- 1 tbsp freshly ground and dried garlic
- 4 fresh tuna steaks, each 1 inch thick

Procedure

First turn on the grill to a high heat. Take the tune fish steaks and brush on the oil. Turn the steaks around and brush some more oil. Sprinkle each steak with salt and pepper.

Place the tuna fish steaks into the grill and ensure that you grill each side for about 2 ½ minutes only. Make sure to turn the other side once done. Remember to leave the center raw otherwise the tune will become dry and tough. Let the steaks rest for about 5 minutes and serve.

9. Grilled Beef Tenderloin

Ingredients

- o   2 tbsp animal or fish oil
- o   2 tsp coarse sea salt
- o   4 beef fillet pieces, 6 to 8 ounces each
- o   Freshly ground black pepper

Preparation

Take the beef fillet pieces from the refrigerator about a half hour before cooking. Turn on the grill to medium heat. Place the beef fillets in a bowl and apply the oil lightly using a brush. Pour some salt and seasoning on the beef fillets to taste.

Now place them on the grill for a bout 4 minutes without turning until grill marks begin to appear. Turn on the beef fillets and let them cook for a further 4 to 5 minutes. The beef fillets are now ready to serve. You can enjoy the delicious meat with a sauce of choice. Bone broth would be great in this instance or a beef stew.

10. Spicy Chicken Stew

Ingredients

- 2 tbsp dried freshly ground red pepper
- 2 tbsp freshly ground black pepper
- 1 tbsp coriander seeds
- 1 tbsp cumin seeds
- 2 tbsp coarse sea salt
- Tender chicken cut up into pieces
- 1 tbsp dried spices
- ½ cup warm water

Procedure

Take the chicken pieces and place them in the bowl. Add some spices and seasoning. Let the chicken sit and marinate for about 15 minutes. Put a large saucepan on medium heat on the stove. Pour in the oil and add the chicken pieces.

Turn the heat to low and cover the sauce pan. Let the chicken cook for a couple of minutes. Open the pan and season the chicken with the red pepper, black pepper, and salt. Cover the pan and let the chicken continue to cook. After 10 minutes, open the pan and pour in a little warm water.

Cover the pan and let the stew simmer. Taste the stew and add some salt, seasoning, or pepper to taste. Allow it to simmer for a further five minutes. If the stew is thick enough and sufficiently seasoned, remove from the stove and set aside.

Your chicken stew is now ready to serve. It should have a nice, tasty, thick stew which you can pour into a cup. Enjoy your delicious spicy chicken and the thick stew.

Carnivore Snacks

1. Boiled eggs

Take some eggs and add them to boiling water. Boil the eggs for 3 to 8 minutes depending on how you like them. 3 minutes for soft boiled and 5 to 8 minutes for hard boiled. Remove the shell then add some salt to taste.

2. Chicken nuggets

Simply take some chicken pieces, season with your favorite seasoning and grill for a couple of minutes on medium heat.

3. Sunnyside up egg

You will need an egg and salt. Simply fry an egg using a shallow pan. Just fry one side without breaking the yolk. Season the egg with salt and pepper and then transfer to a plate.

4. Fried chicken entrails

Simply fry chicken entrails on a pan. Add some oil and seasoning. Cook for 3 to 5 minutes only.

5. Left over beef chunks

You can warm some left over beef chunks and have them for a mid-morning or afternoon snack

6. Bacon slices

Season some bacon and fry them on a shallow frying pan on low heat

7. Beef sausages

Boil some beef sausages then season before frying on a shallow skillet

8. Fish fingers

Fish fingers are easy to prepare. You can buy them at the grocery store and simply cook them on a skillet on low heat for a few minutes

9. Meat balls

Meatballs are easy to prepare. Mince your preferred meat and season it then mould into spherical shape. Grill in the oven for 10 - 15 minutes.

10. Prawns

Prepare prawns and season them appropriately. Have them for your evening snack

Chapter Six

Benefits of the Carnivore Diet

Major benefits of the carnivore diet

It reduces inflammation

The carnivore diet has many benefits. It is considered as the lead anti-inflammatory diet for patients suffering autoimmune conditions. It also has numerous other health benefits.

This diet lowers your insulin levels significantly. Anyone suffering from insulin-related challenges like diabetes will benefit from lower insulin levels. Some patients have testified of getting cured of diabetes.

Simple eating method

The carnivore diet provides a simple way of eating. Dieters pursuing this way of eating do not have to count calories or eat at certain times. This diet requires you to eat as much as you can whenever you want. You eat to satisfaction without any concern and will still lose weight.
Some people worry about counting calories, meal preparations, and macronutrients, and so on. ***All these worries are fortunately not valid with the carnivore diet.***

Your digestive system will improve

While there is no fiber associated with the carnivore diet, it does promote a healthy digestive system. There is reason to believe that cutting fiber from your diet actually improves your digestive system.

Improved mental clarity

You will enjoy improved mental clarity just like those on the keto diet do. Our brains are made up of 60% fat so a diet with plenty of fat will support the brain. Experts attribute improved mental clarity to restricted carbs intake with increase protein and fat intake.

Reduced inflammation

According to a 3-month study by health practitioners in the US state of Georgia, it was established that persons on a low carb, high fat diet had lower inflammation levels in general compared to those on a high carb, low fat diet.

Faster weight loss

Despite common presumption, you will actually lose weight faster on the carnivore diet. The body usually accumulates fat because it is not insulin sensitive. This means that any time you consume carbs, they are converted into fat. However, if you completely cut out carbs from your diet, your body will become extremely sensitive to insulin. Your hunger hormones are regulated so that you do not eat unnecessarily.

Improves testosterone levels

High fat diets have been shown to improve testosterone levels. It is known that testosterone levels tend to decrease with age. This is a situation that can be changed and turned around through the high fat, high protein diet.

It helps improve condition of patients with autoimmune conditions

Plenty of patients with autoimmune conditions like MS have seen their symptoms improve drastically by practicing and following the carnivore diet. It is also great for patients with chronic conditions like high blood pressure and diabetes.

It cleanses and detoxifies the body

By taking the carnivore diet, you will help to cleanse your body and eliminate toxins.

Worthwhile lifestyle to pursue

To many people, the carnivore diet sounds a little crazy. They think it is a highly risky and deficient diet that will harm the body. This is actually not true. There are numerous anecdotal testaments of people who have experienced significant weight loss, increased mental focus, and improved health and mood markers that make it hard to ignore the diet.

A diet that restricts the consumption of unnecessary calories especially from carbs will definitely benefit your body. You will actually lose weight while enjoying a juicy steak and delicious ribs.

Intermittent Fasting and the Carnivore Diet

Intermittent fasting is a lifestyle that requires you to fast for a period of time then have your meals during another much smaller window. You will generally fast for much longer with an eating window of only a few hours.

While the carnivore diet dictates that you eat as much as you can whenever you want, intermittent fasting calls for alternate periods of fasting and eating. However, it is possible to incorporate intermittent fasting with your all-meat diet.

The good news is that it is possible to follow an intermittent fasting lifestyle with the carnivore diet. **This is because meat is very satisfying so you are able to go for lengthy periods of time without eating.**

Intermittent fasting does not dictate the foods that you eat but only provides eating and fasting windows. Therefore, during your eating windows you will strictly adhere to the carnivore diet.

What to Expect with Intermittent Fasting

- You can expect to lose lots of weight, much more than you would on a normal diet
- You will not feel hungry regularly as you would on a regular diet
- Most of your cravings will disappear
- Your allergies will also disappear with time
- Expect to have a clear head
- Your body will be more efficient in cleansing and detoxification

Conclusion

The next step is to begin following this diet as instructed. You can do this slowly- following one step at a time. The best level to begin at is level one. Follow the instructions provided and proceed all the way to level three.

Within a few short weeks or months, you will begin to enjoy the numerous benefits of this diet. Your initial challenges will eventually disappear and you will begin to feel great. You will also be in a great position to heal your body and see all the symptoms of any chronic conditions disappear.

Subscribe to our Carnivore Diet blog at:

www.CarnivoreCleanse.com

References

Health.com
https://www.health.com/nutrition/carnivore-diet

Meat Health
https://meat.health/knowledge-base/carnivore-diet-what-to-eat/

Everyday Health
https://www.everydayhealth.com/diet-nutrition/diet/carnivore-diet-benefits-risks-food-list-more/

ONNIT Academy
https://www.onnit.com/academy/the-carnivore-diet/

Book Two

Intermittent Fasting

Burn Fat, Lose Weight,
Become Energetic and Happy

*Use The Power Of Your Body To Lose
Weight and Increase Health*

Michael D Kaiser

Table of Contents

Chapter One	94
The History of Fasting	94
Chapter Two	99
What is Wrong With Our Modern Diets?	99
Chapter Three	105
The Science of How it Works	105
Chapter Four	112
Keys to Success	112
Chapter Five	117
Chapter Six	121
Three Meals a Day is a Social Construct.	121
Chapter Seven	124
Established Intermittent Meal Plans	124
Chapter Eight	127
Training and Fasting	127
Chapter Nine	131
What Foods Can You Eat	131
Chapter Ten	138
Sample Meal Ideas	138
Additional Resources	141
Conclusion	142

Introduction

The world of dieting is growing increasingly chaotic. People are confused as to what "diet" will work and what foods are safe to eat, even healthy foods. This has led to the creation of prehistoric diets that are trying to model what a caveman or pre-historic man/woman ate, as that should be the most optimal diet for humans today. Although it works for many people, we are not cave people anymore nor are we spending 15 hours a day hunting and gathering food just to survive.

The other problem facing so many people today is that we have so much rich food available to us everywhere we go, it constantly surrounds us and is easily available. Most of the food is processed or infused with chemicals that cause it to not be digested properly which drains our energy during the day, making it difficult to focus or work.

I personally simply use a mostly vegetarian whole foods diet in my daily intermittent fasting, even though I have tried many other diets and foods, I found that the whole foods works best for me, in intermittent fasting, which includes 2-3 weekly servings of healthy fish, chicken or beef. It wasn't until I started intermittent fasting that I saw amazing results. At first I thought it was my diet or maybe the sprints I was doing, or the supplement I was taking, but no, it was fasting for 15-16 hours a day that was making the changes.

The biggest change was the reduction of what little sub-cutaneous fat I still had, so that my abs were finally visible, and my veins became visible too. Then the biomarkers in my blood increased, and when I became very strict about eating only whole natural foods with no added oils, sugar or other chemicals that disrupt the body, things really became amazing. Today I often get comments that I appear to be in my early thirties or even late twenties, and I am 41 years old as of this writing. I attribute a lot of the health benefits to INTERMITTENT FASTING, but for optimal health it is really going to be many factors (food choices, exercise, attitude, sun exposure, genetics, etc.)

This book is a basic introductory to Intermittent Fasting for the beginner

It will get you started with the following basics:

- What Intermittent Fasting is and how it works.
- What popular Intermittent Fasting diets are on the market now.
- How to customize one that works for you and your lifestyle.
- How to integrate it into your life so that it becomes a habit and not a "diet"

The first step will not always be the easiest, which is why the information you will find in the following chapters is so important to take to heart, as they are concepts that can be put into action immediately.

I personally started my own intermittent fasting program in 2015 and it was what ended my plateau I found myself in. I was already very athletic and trying to eat healthy. I permanently lost an additional 12 pounds of fat from intermittent fasting for only a few months. I was already in great shape, ran, jogged, sprinted and cycled almost daily. The biggest discovery I made from intermittent fasting is that I get full really fast when I do eat, so I really do not eat that much. You will probably discover the same effect. More importantly, the biggest benefit I received for fasting daily is the health benefits I feel, the less I ate all the time, the better I felt. It was very strange, but I realized that when I WASN'T eating, I felt great. That's when I discovered that eating through-out the day is not for me anymore, and is more of a strain than anything else.

The following chapters will discuss the preparedness you will need to really lose weight and gain the health benefits of intermittent fasting. This means that you will want to consider the quality of your food, including the potential issues raised by their quality, how they can best be utilized in a meal, as well as various tools you might need to keep your mind focused on the task at hand.

Chapter One

The History of Fasting

The intermittent fasting diet, invented by Ori Hofmekler, is based on a daily food cycle that includes two phases: underfeeding during the day and overfeeding during the evening-night.

The phase of underfeeding should last all day, applying the rules of the intermittent fasting diet. This naturally stimulates the sympathetic nervous system (SNS) which promotes vigilance, competitiveness, and energy expenditure. During this time, the body moves into a negative energy balance and is therefore forced to burn stored fat to produce energy.

During the underfeeding phase, the consumption of food consisting mostly of raw fruits and vegetables, soups, and small amounts of protein foods should be minimized.

The major food intake phase takes place during the evening-night hours.

This is the moment when the main meal should be consumed when you can eat as much as you want from all the food groups but still following certain dietary patterns, which we will dwell on more later.

Physically active individuals may require more energy and special types of fuel (fats or carbohydrates), depending on the nature and level of their physical activity. The phase of food abundance causes the activation of the parasympathetic nervous system (SNP), which promotes relaxation and recovery.

During this phase, the body moves towards a positive energy balance while creating a general anabolic-constructive state. This is the moment when the body recovers, builds the tissues and fills the energy reserves.

An example of Intermittent fasting were the soldiers of the Roman Empire who were subjected to major stresses for wars and large displacements. They were trained to fight and possessed powerful bodies and important muscle masses, so they carried a lot of energy accumulated in the periods of rest.

More specifically, the Hofmekler model, which also partly refers to intermittent fasting and caloric restriction studies, provides only one large meal a day after 10-12 hours of fasting or limited to the intake of small protein snacks or fruit or vegetable juices.

Under these conditions, the organism would interpret the fast as a sort of state of emergency and consequently synthesize a whole series of hormones that favor the transformation of fats into energy (growth hormone, adrenaline, noradrenaline) and improve the physical response to the environmental circumstances.

According to Hofmekler, the fact that breakfast is considered the most important meal of the day has no scientific basis, while the human body would be more alert and efficient if you keep fasting until evening.

Man is, by nature, a nocturnal eater programmed to work and fast during the day and eat and rest during the night, while it would be customary to consume his meals during the day which, going against nature, promotes the development of obesity, diabetes, heart attack and stroke.

During the day, you will have to eat completely natural foods, such as vegetables, a little fruit, and small amounts of protein.

The goal of the intermittent fasting diet is to create a lifestyle that imitates that of our predecessors from prehistory to ancient Rome (primitives and gladiators).

To summarize everything, we could say that this food model is based on the assumption that nourishing the body by supporting the circadian rhythms of primitive man is functional to the maintenance of physical form and health, as it enhances the use of nutrients and the transformation of body fat into energy while at the same time increasing resistance to stress.

The author has "engraved" the real commandments that "the warrior" subjected to this diet will have to follow. Those are:

- Provide your body with all the essential nutrients (vitamins, minerals, EFA, amino acids, and probiotics). Introduce all the aromas, flavors, textures and colors possible.

- When possible, cyclically rotate the days when carbohydrates, proteins, or fats dominate the caloric percentages taken.

- Avoid foods containing hormones, pesticides, chemical additives, sugar alcohols, artificial sweeteners, and excess fructose.

- Do not eat foods that contain high-glycemic carbohydrates on their own.

- Exercise regularly even during the underfeeding phase.

Avoid wrong food combinations such as:

- Wheat and sugar
- Starch and fats
- Walnuts and parmesan
- Carbohydrates and alcohol

The body is designed to eat this way.

The cyclicity between negative energetic and positive energy balance of genes known as "parsimonious genes" improves human survival chances. This is measured by the ability to improve energy use, performance, and health. Intermittent fasting lets you turn on biological switches that improve human survival day by day.

In the morning, just wake up, and on an empty stomach, we have 3 main substances in circulation:

- testosterone – every man has a peak of it in the morning;
- cortisol – a stress hormone, extremely lipolytic hormone;
- catecholamines — adrenaline and noradrenaline, pure energy.

All these hormones increase energy aggression and mental clarity, and they are stimulated by the empty stomach.

In this fasting phase, you will lose weight and water.

If you start eating at this stage of the day, you would raise insulin and GH—hormones that make you calm, relaxed but little aggressive, lazy, feel weak, and immediately store the energies and lower the 3 hormones above.

The blood then moves away from the muscles to go to the stomach for digestion and therefore less blood to the muscles.

Another positive outcome from fasting is its purification effect on the liver and the kidney.

In the overeating phase, you have to start eating less tasty foods and then move on to tastier foods, so you will start with the intake of salad, vegetables, proteins—then finish with the richest carbohydrate foods.

> It will be important to introduce a wide variety of foods—both from the point of view of flavor, consistency and color—to get all the nutritive principles (macro and micronutrients).

Chapter Two

What is Wrong With Our Modern Diets?

Have you ever wondered why we eat? It is one of those simple questions behind our discovery of the complex mechanisms that run our lives. The first reason why we eat is that it allows us to grow from being an infant until we reach our maturity as an adult. The second function of nutrition is to conserve life. Food gives energy to our body and maintains a caloric level sufficient to conserve the temperature of the body of each species. In this case, human beings have a normal body temperature of 37 degrees Celsius.

What happens if food is not consumed? The body takes calories from the fat tissue, which is temporarily stored mostly in your belly when you eat. A good health refers to keeping the process of food input and food expenditure in balance. If you eat too much, you go beyond the natural purpose for which fat deposits exist. This will make you obese.

In the richest countries, obesity is an increasingly widespread phenomenon. Various explanations are given as to why there is a widespread obesity in such countries. For some, the impulse to eat beyond measure comes from an ancestral hunger, sort of a command left in the brain and ready to be activated in the presence of food.

For others, the explanation is psychological. In fact, we create an abnormal situation with this almost neurotic need for excessive nutrition. Just look at how many mothers overfeed their children today.

Positive food education

Today, everything is turned upside down, and it is often the children who blackmail their parents by threatening not to eat if they do not turn up the television or condescend to their desires. Instead, the golden rule is to eat little. Not only because of the cardiovascular risks related to being overweight, but also because more food is introduced, and more risks are incurred for cancer. The risk of cancer is proportional to the amount of food that is introduced: more food, more risks. This is why I decided to write this book: to make an invitation to frugality and, maybe, to inspire parents to be stricter with their children.

Many food pathologies are linked to a culture that has lost sight of what really is necessary to survive. Diseases such as anorexia and bulimia did not exist almost 30-40 years ago when there was education in food and attention to its good use. As Bismarck said, you can forget the rules of healthy eating on your birthday, but you do not have to celebrate your birthday every day.

Even this apparently simple question proposes to our attention the mechanism of life on Earth and its conservation and propagation. It is a complex alchemy, which occurs in a regime of mutual exchange between those that our elementary school books defined, with a suggestive word, the "kingdoms of nature—" mineral, vegetable, and animal. The plant world absorbs carbon dioxide from the atmosphere and transforms it into plants, which, in turn, produce oxygen.

The animal world behaves in an opposite way and is the protagonist of a reverse project: it absorbs oxygen and burns it, producing carbon dioxide. The Earth lives on this harmonious relationship: on the one hand, plants produce what animals consume, and the product of this process serves the vegetable world to live.

And now, let's go back to the history of man. Man is a primate, which means that he is a modified monkey, and the monkey has maintained very basic metabolic characteristics. Primates have been and still are vegetarians and also interact with the plant world because they basically eat fruit.

The flowers, from which the fruit will then be born, are colored and fragrant because they have to attract pollinating insects that allow fertilization. The fruits, equally colored and fragrant, attract animals, including humans. However, this harmony and this synergy between different kingdoms and worlds at some point in human history started to suffer from a great problem: the great glaciations. The plants disappeared almost completely. Many vegetarian animals perished miserably.

The human species was saved, and from a vegetarian species became a carnivore one. The turning point of human nutrition was the ice that covered the planet. Men became carnivorous, but also maintained the metabolism of a vegetarian primate. In short, our organism is programmed for the consumption of fruit and vegetables, and to return largely to this type of food can only benefit us.

We should follow the example of our ancestors' peasants.

Mediterranean Diet

The so-called Mediterranean diet—based on vegetables, fruit, and pasta—has been proven effective in preventing diseases such as cardiovascular diseases, obesity, diabetes and cancer.

The return to a Mediterranean diet has contributed, together with more effective drugs, to the reduction of mortality from cardiovascular diseases. The Mediterranean diet is the diet that has handed down to us the peasant population of America and of all those countries that overlook the Mediterranean Sea. You ate a little meat, a lot of fish (if you lived on the shores of the sea), cereals, pasta, legumes, vegetables, and fruits. It was a poor but balanced diet, and it was enough to sustain life.

The situation today is a tragic paradox; on one side, there is the poor world starving; on the other, the rich world dying of obesity.

What is intermittent fasting?

Although it may seem absurd, fasting is good for the mind and the body. There are many forms of "the fasting diet," but the type that has been rediscovered in recent times is that of intermittent fasting.

The diet varies: from allowing the consumption of calories only for a certain period of the day (usually from six to twelve hours) to drastic caloric reduction for 48 hours—until complete fasting every week.

The studies on intermittent fasting are innumerable, many of which are still "work in progress," but significant benefits are being highlighted on several aspects.

In addition to losing weight, intermittent fasting would also improve blood pressure and help the body dispose of fat by going into ketosis.

Positive indicators also seem to be related to the reduction of cancer risk, especially breast cancer—yet they are still in progress.

Returning to weight, it has been proven that the more the body accuses the fast, the more it uses fat as fuel, thus entering into ketosis.

Not only that: there would be a positive feedback as well regarding a significant reinforcement of neural connections with consequent improvement of memory and mood.

Those who practice intermittent fasting report feeling more lucid and focused during fasting.

Scientists would argue that ketogenic diets would help to fight diseases like Alzheimer's - precisely because of this cognitive improvement at the hands of fasting, which also improves mood.

Intermittent fasting would seem to be propaedeutic even for diabetes.

A fast that includes, for example, a few days without particular restrictions on food—always following a healthy and controlled diet—followed by a very narrow diet of 5 days, would bring significant improvements to those with high blood sugar.

Prof. Valter Longo is considered the guru of food and anti-aging, and his studies on human aging have led him to develop the Diet Mima Fasting (another type of fasting diet).

DMF is able to give the healthy and anti-aging benefits of fasting while at the same time eating normally the remaining twenty-five days a month.

It is not certain that intermittent fasting can bring about the same benefits, even if it is possible.

Professor Longo's recommendation is not to abuse the term "intermittent fasting."

It is known that some forms of fasting—how to consistently restrict food during one or two days a week or eat only at certain times—bring health benefits, but it is not yet known whether this applies to all types of fasting.

Chapter Three

The Science of How it Works

Before getting into the details of intermittent fasting, I'd like to spend some time talking about the basics of nutrition. When we talk about diet and nutrition, we often do not know the principles that underlie our very existence and, above all, our physical well-being. We limit ourselves to eating something that others have advised us, and we often take pills and tablets advertised, which not only have no use but wrapped up can even be harmful to our health and our finances.

In order not to get lost in the sea of nutrition, the first useful thing is to make an overview of food principles and daily human needs.

Let's start by saying that all foods can be classified into five large food groups:
- carbohydrates
- proteins (or protides)
- fats (or lipids)
- vitamins
- minerals

Carbohydrates are the elements most present in our diet. They are made up of two main elements—carbon and water—that when joined together give rise to the simplest of sugars, glucose. Aggregating then into larger molecules, they form two different groups of carbohydrates: simple sugars (consisting of a few molecules of glucose) and complex sugars (formed by long chains of glucose). A subsequent classification is that which divides them into monosaccharides (a sugar molecule), disaccharides (two molecules), and polysaccharides (more than two molecules).

There are about 200 different types of carbohydrates, and oftentimes, they take the name from the food in which they are in large quantities. For instance, there are some carbohydrates called fructose, lactose, maltose, but also sucrose and starch. Carbohydrates are mainly from vegetables, and their function is purely energetic and makes up the basis of human nutrition—providing about 4 calories per gram/weight. They are found in large quantities in pasta, rice, potatoes, fruit, bread, flour as well as in legumes.

The cells of our body transform all the carbohydrates introduced into the simplest form, glycogen, which, once oxidized into the cellular mitochondria, provides energy for rapid and above-all clean use, i.e. without waste. These must, therefore, represent the basis of our nutrition and must provide about 60-65% of the energy needs.

However, it is rare to have to carry out a glucosidic supplementation. In fact, they are so widely present in all foods, that perhaps we should think about reducing their consumption.

Fats, on the other hand, are complex acidic structures found in both animal and vegetable foods. Like carbohydrates, fats also have a purely energetic function, with a different caloric value. Lipids bring about 9 calories per gram/weight, and their burning rate is very slow. In fact, before being used, fats must be transformed into simpler elements, which the cell can then oxidize to obtain energy. In their complex form, on the other hand, they are easily stored as fat storage, which is the energy reserve of our body. Fats are often divided into saturated and unsaturated, depending on the type of chemical bond that forms the molecule. To simplify, we can say that saturated fats are "bad" **and harmful to our arteries**—these include cholesterol, glycerol, hydrogenated fats, fats contained in butter and margarine, palm oil, and most fats of animal origin.

The "good" fats instead are the unsaturated fats or those contained in nuts, avocados and fish fats (omega 3 and omega 6), and lecithin (abundant in soybeans).

In addition to energy capacity, fats are involved in many organic activities, including hormone synthesis and cell membrane construction. Their function is therefore vital, and our energy needs should be covered by lipids in the measure of 15-20%.

The integration of fats is very rare, as we usually tend to consume more than we should since they are the vehicle of taste and make us better appreciate the foods we ingest.

When it comes to proteins, it is a totally different story. They are composed of complex chains of amino acids joined together by peptide bonds. These amino acids can bind together in number, proportions, and different forms—giving rise to an almost infinite series of specific proteins.

There are 21 amino acids, 8 of which are called "essential," because our body is not able to synthesize them. In fact, human RNA possesses protein synthesis codes for only 13 amino acids and is able to process proteins that contain only these elements. For a complete protein range, it is necessary to take the remaining 8 amino acids, called essential amino acids, from the outside through eating.

Animal and vegetable proteins are made of the same amino acids—with a substantial difference. While each animal protein contains all 21 amino acids (in different proportions, depending on the protein itself), in the proteins coming from vegetables, there is always something missing. Some plant foods, therefore, contain certain amino acids but do not contain others. It becomes important, then, in the case of a vegetarian diet, to know how to combine the various products so that all the necessary elements are introduced. As we said, this does not apply to animal proteins, which are called "noble" because they are complete.

From an energetic point of view, protides are similar to carbohydrates, bringing about 4 calories per gram/weight. Unfortunately, the energy obtained from proteins is not as clean, because as a result of oxidation at the cellular level, nitrogen is released, which then evolves into free radicals, accelerating the cellular aging process.

The energetic process of proteins is just a *fallback* of the body in the event of an actual need for calories. Normally, protides are used for "plastic" purposes, i.e. they are used in the construction, repair, and renewal of all body structures—such as muscles, bones, cells, organs, apparatuses, and tissues, in general. It can be said that the human body is composed of 70% water, and the rest of it is proteins. To maintain itself, the human body, therefore, needs a certain daily protein intake, which should be about one gram per kilogram of body weight (a man of 80 kilograms should take 80 grams of protein per day). However, this proportion can range between 0.70 grams per kilogram/weight (the minimum to remain healthy) up to a maximum of 1.5 grams per kilogram/weight. Beyond this threshold, you risk that the proteins are used for energetic purposes would rise to many free radicals and other problems related to kidneys and liver. Ultimately, the daily heat intake of proteins should be 15-20%.

The integration of proteins may be necessary in the case of a vegetarian diet, while it's not recommended in a varied diet, including animal foods. Moreover, the assimilation of protides for plastic use is about 4 grams per hour, so we can assume that the body has more means of using them for energy. However, the proteins taken through supplements are less similar than those taken through normal nutrition, as they are metabolized with a certain amount of carbohydrates and vitamins (especially B12).

Another important part of nutrition is the macro group of vitamins. They are organic compounds essential to life and development that normally the human body cannot synthesize and must, therefore, take with food. They are found in large quantities in vegetables and fruits. Many vitamins are sensitive to high temperatures, so it is advisable to take these foods raw. Moreover, some of them deteriorate over time, becoming bioavailable—this is why it is preferable to eat freshly picked fruits and vegetables.

Each vitamin has a specific function, which can vary from the metabolic one (e.g. B12) to the protective one of the blood vessels (vitamin C). The deficiency of a certain vitamin, usually called avitaminosis, can cause specific diseases, such as scurvy in the case of vitamin C deficiency.

Vitamins are distinguished between two categories: water-soluble ones (which means they can be melted in water) and liposoluble ones (melted in fats). Our body is able to store the fat-soluble vitamins (A, D, E, K, and F), while it cannot retain the water-soluble vitamins (C, B1, B2, B5, B6, B12, H, PP) that are easily eliminated in the urine. The latter, in fact, should be taken several times throughout the day. It is also worthy to note that fat-soluble vitamins, which are stored in body fat, have a slower process of elimination. This can cause, in the case of a high intake, a state of toxicity, thus creating very serious dysfunctions. Therefore, if an integration of water-soluble vitamins can be made lightly, we must instead pay maximum attention when it comes to the fat-soluble ones, which should be integrated only in case of established deficiency.

The last food group is one of the minerals and inorganic elements (i.e. without biological carbon) that cover multiple functions. They are often called mineral salts, but this is an improper name since most minerals are devoid of the salt part. Rather, they are single elements present in nature—metals and non-metals—which use water as a vehicle to pass from the earth to the plants and therefore to the animals that feed on them.

They are divided into three groups: macro-elements, micro-elements, and oligo-elements. This division is established on the basis of the daily requirement of the elements, which can vary from 100 milligrams/day for the macro-elements (calcium, phosphorus, potassium, etc.), to less than 200 micrograms/day for the oligo-elements (manganese, chromium, cobalt, etc.).

Although their presence in the body is around 5%/6% of the body weight, they are of vital importance, as they participate in many cellular and metabolic functions. Just think, for instance, about iron, which plays an important part in the cardiovascular system; or calcium, which is a fundamental element of bones and teeth. They must, therefore, be eaten on a regular basis, as the body expels them through the excretory apparatus through urine, feces, and sweat.

A varied diet in which vegetables, fruit, meat, fish, eggs, and dried fruit are added, provides the optimal amount of all the necessary minerals.

Mineral deficiency, just like vitamins, can lead to specific diseases, such as iron deficiency anemia, or it can even aggravate diseases such as osteoporosis in the case of calcium deficiency. A certain quantity of minerals is therefore vital, but their excess can instead lead to real phenomena of poisoning. Hence, it would be good to stay away from the saline and mineral supplements, unless there's an ascertained shortage. Most importantly, before starting the intake through supplements, it is advisable to seek medical advice.

Chapter Four

Keys to Success

Tips and Tricks with Intermittent Fasting

The idea of starting a diet can be daunting, especially if you are not mentally prepared to face such a change. When the mind is calm and prepared, sticking to a healthy food program is much simpler. With the right preparation, you will be able to effectively achieve your goals, and you will make it less difficult not to fall into temptation during the journey.

Be aware of the recurring negative thoughts related to food.

Oftentimes, our diets fail because of our beliefs related to food and eating. Try to become aware of your food beliefs and make an effort to change your mentality.

We often think that on special occasions, it is ok to let go a bit. There's nothing wrong with eating a little more from time to time, but be honest with yourself about what you consider "special occasions." When events like eating away from home, business lunches, office parties, and other small events all become excuses to let yourself binge, the failure of the diet is just around the corner. Try, therefore, to re-evaluate what occasions can be considered as "special" and when it is better to stick to your original diet plan.

Do you use food as a reward?

Many think that after a long busy day, it is normal to deserve to go out for dinner or eat an entire tub of ice cream. Look for alternative ways to reward yourself, which do not include food. For example, take a long hot bath, buy a new dress, or go to the cinema. There are many ways to reward yourself without using food.

The importance of listening to your body

Dissociate food from certain activities.

Food is closely linked to numerous rituals. Giving up sugar and fat may not be easy when we emotionally associate them with certain habits. Make a conscious effort to break these dangerous associations.

Try to be aware of the times you eat too much or make bad food choices, both in terms of food and the things you drink. Whenever you go to the cinema, do you buy Coca-Cola and popcorn? Cannot say "no" to a few glasses of wine during the evenings out? Cannot imagine a Saturday morning without coffee and donuts? If so, take the extra mile to commit to chopping these associations.

Try changing associations by replacing harmful foods with healthier ones. For example, when you spend the evening out, dedicate it to a board game instead of focusing on drinking. On Saturday mornings, have breakfast with coffee, yogurt, and fresh fruits. If, at the end of the day, you tend to try to relax through eating, replace the food with a good book or some music.

It is not just about calories.

In the end, you will be more likely to be able to stick to your diet by committing yourself to change your negative behaviors rather than just keeping your calories under control. Try to become aware of when you eat and why you do it. Even if it is only half a biscuit, ask yourself if you are allowing it because you think you have had a bad day. Do you tend to eat because you are hungry or because you feel bored? If you do it out of boredom, try to get rid of this bad habit. Even if you do not exceed the calories, always try to use common sense. Do not eat the wrong foods for the wrong reasons.

Ask for help.

Changing is not easy, and sometimes, we are not able to do it on our own. Ask for help from friends and family. Let them know you are trying to lose weight, and pray to support yourself. Make sure they know they do not have to invite you to parties where cheap food and alcohol will be served. In addition, ask to be able to vent with them in moments when you will feel particularly frustrated or tempted. Share your goals with all the people living under your own roof.

Establish contained and realistic goals.

Many people tend to sabotage their diet by placing the bar of expectations too high. If you want to be able to stick to your plans, set goals achievable.

Remember that a balanced diet allows you to lose about ½-1 kilo a week, no more. If you intend to lose weight faster than that, prepare to fail.

Initially, you should have cautious goals, so you will be more likely to be able to reach them and have the motivation to continue. Unspecific intentions, such as "This week, I will eat vegetables every day," and something like, "The next time I eat out of the house, I will order a salad instead of potato chips," are valid starting points that can lead you to the road to success.

Keep a diary.

If you want your diet to be successful, you cannot exempt yourself from being responsible. Go out and buy a diary that will accompany you along the entire route. Record everything you eat every day, and keep a calorie count. A tangible account will force you to notice your bad habits and motivate you to develop new ones.

Plan your meals.

Planning meals and snacks in advance will help you not to give in to temptations. In the days before the start of the diet, make a list of healthy recipes that you intend to prepare. Try to get ahead, for example, by buying or cutting the necessary ingredients. If you want, you can also cook soups and vegetables to keep in the refrigerator—they will be very useful for the first week lunches.

Focus on concrete behavior.

Limiting yourself to making analyses in abstract terms, it will not be easy to develop greater willpower. Examining your concrete actions will help you start the transformation.
Make a list of the wrong habits you want to change. Start with small, gradual changes. Try to commit yourself to abandon an old behavior for a week, then continue making new changes slowly.

For example, you decide that after work, rather than watching a show, you will walk for 40 minutes. Commit to respecting your purpose for a week. In the following days, you can gradually increase the duration of the exercise, e.g. by walking for an hour.

On the occasions when the willpower is not yet sufficient, commit to bringing yourself back to the right path, even if it may mean having to be particularly hard on yourself. Doing so will help you understand that you are the only one who has the power to change your behavior.

Recognize and admit any failures. Register them on your food diary. Take responsibility for failure.

Describe the reasons that led to failure, highlighting your disappointment. For example, write something like, "At dinner, I ate dessert because I chose to, and I felt guilty after doing it." Although they may sound harsh words, many believe that saying them is useful to express clearly that they have failed. You will feel motivated to make greater efforts to be able to change.

For some, taking a weekly meal "out of the rules" can be a valid help to stay on track. A deprivation that has lasted too long may cause the whole project to go up in smoke. Sticking to a strict diet may seem more feasible when you know that at the end of the tunnel, you can give yourself the coveted food. If you think it might be useful to check you, consider scheduling a premium meal at the end of the week.

Chapter Five

Common Questions

Eating is a necessary activity—the body is like a car, and without fuel, it cannot work. Unfortunately, however, in our society, overloaded with food and obsessed with dieting, people build a relationship with extremely wrong foods, in which the act of eating becomes an automatic action and too often linked to negative emotions. In this chapter, I will try to explain to you what is the only thing you need to do to improve your relationship with food and make the act of eating an action that will not only bring nourishment but also pleasure.

Have you ever eaten food without even knowing what they are?

Do not worry; unfortunately, it happens to many people. Every day, people come to my studio to tell me how they respond unconsciously to their food stimuli, always repeating the same actions and, above all, feeling deprived of the strength to change.

They tell me how often they do not derive any joy from what they eat and, on the contrary, gain a lot of frustration or guilt from it, and they want to know what they can do to improve their relationship with food. They have often tried everything and feel tired and disappointed.

The solution is actually much simpler than what you may believe.

The only thing you need to do to improve your relationship

with food is not to do stressful diets (which only lower self-esteem) or spend whole days in the gym, but something much simpler: you have to become more aware of what you are doing.

Increasing awareness of your automated models can help you make more deliberate food choices and improve your relationship with food.

What you have to change is not so much the food you eat, but more on our relationship with it. Learning to eat with awareness will allow you to understand what your body really needs, and it will allow you to enjoy your meals.

In this way, in the end, you will reach your ideal weight without having to constantly resort to exasperating diets.

How do you do it?

Simple: you have to learn to be in contact with *you*! You have to ask yourself some good questions to help you become aware of the hundreds of food decisions you take every day without even realizing it.

Here are some good questions you must ask yourself to become more aware and improve your relationship with food.

1. Why do I eat?

This is the main question that will guide all your future decisions. And in the vast majority of cases, you do not know why you're eating! People hardly stop to wonder what drives them to go to the kitchen and open the pantry drawer. Many times, one believes that they are hungry, but in reality, they only feel like that in response to an emotional stimulus, such as boredom or stress. Learning to recognize this difference is the first step to effectively fight your urges and discover the real needs of your body. Take a break to ask yourself, "Am I really hungry?" Whenever you feel like you need to eat, it will help you differentiate your physical hunger from environmental and emotional stimuli.

2. When do I eat?

If you have ever followed a diet in your life, you will have realized that the traditional dietary approaches do nothing but provide you with a food plan where they tell you what you should eat, how much you have to eat, and what time you have to eat! This cannot be more wrong. These rules do nothing but disconnect you from your natural nourishment needs and only encourage you to ignore internal signals of hunger and satiety.

3. What do I eat?

Diets are definitely frustrating. They force you to eliminate a lot of things and often the best ones in terms of taste! To be able to do this, you are required a certain willpower that must be maintained for a very long time, which is very difficult even for the most persevering people. Learning to consume a little of everything in a moderate way, ranging from healthier foods to those that you eat for pleasure, will lead you to live your relationship with food in a much more balanced way. By freeing yourself from restrictions, you will develop the ability to respond to the wisdom of your body—that innate wisdom that is within each person.

4. How do I eat?

Quickly? Standing up? Watching TV? Many people eat this way and are so inclined to eat more—this feeling of satiety and satisfaction is, in fact, less when not paying attention to the food you introduce. Learn to avoid multitasking when you eat and dedicate quality time to the activity of eating. In this way, you will be able to feel what your body has to tell you, such as when it is time to stop, so as to avoid the binge you will later regret.

5. How much do you eat?

Normally, classic diets focus on how much you are allowed to eat using methods based on the control of calories or fat. This behavior, however, in the long run, leads you to spend an enormous amount of time, energy, and willpower. Turning the meal into a mechanical experience will make you disconnect from internal signals, and this will favor problematic behaviors rather than reducing them. Paying attention to the signs of satiety and determining small goals in the situation, such as feeling better after eating than before you start, will make you able to eat the "right" amount of food based on the real needs of your body. For example, young children eat when they are hungry and stop when they are full. They touch, smell, and explore food while eating it. Re-learning these innate behaviors in humans is essential for developing a healthy relationship with food.

Chapter Six

Three Meals a Day is a Social Construct.

Why do we eat what we eat? The answer suggested by common sense is that we choose to eat what we like. And it is a correct answer: satisfaction is the main factor influencing our food choices. But the question is more complex. Scientific literature has highlighted a link between food and the expression of both social and personal identity—we are what we eat, not only in biological terms but also in symbolic terms. In fact, food practices refer to the different collective belonging and manifest the individual adherence to a lifestyle. Moreover, social psychology, in explaining human behavior, takes into account the fact that we do not live in isolation but together with other people who inevitably influence us. Therefore, in addition to the tastes and information we possess (for example, on the presumed healthiness of certain foods), the influence of others also contributes to determining our eating habits, often through identification processes with different social groups. Without claiming to be exhaustive, let's look at some examples of social influence on eating behavior.

The first to influence us are certainly our parents, especially our mothers, who can condition us in different ways. First of all, through their example: our mothers are the first models we imitate, in general, and also with regard to the relationship with food. Secondly, our mothers even influence the development of our tastes because it circumscribes and delimits our experience with food: our mothers choose the one that enters the repertoire of the foods we come in contact with and selecting the foods to which we are exposed. When we were in their womb, we began to taste and learn about the flavors of our family and our culture. This selective exposure to food continues throughout the period of breastfeeding (even our mothers' milk takes the taste of what they eat) and continues for a long time. In fact, at least until the children reach 11-12 years old, our parents decide which foods come into the pantry and arrive at the table. This type of influence is fundamental because the selection of the food we are experiencing greatly influences our tastes, which are mainly formed through simple exposure and repeated experience. They are built on familiarity—we like what we are used to eating.

A second way by which tastes develop is through associations that are established between a certain food and a positive or negative situation. Parents can also influence these associations: if the family meal is a nice moment and an opportunity for sharing and living peacefully, our relationship with food will be connoted in a positive sense; if the meal is a battlefield, a place of conflict, in which they force us to eat something that does not go well, then our relationship with food will perhaps be compromised and will haunt us even into adulthood.

Growing up, our peers become increasingly important, both in general and as sources of influence, on our eating behaviour. Our peers influence us because we tend to imitate them. For example, at the end of a dinner with new friends, we often ask ourselves: "Should I get the dessert?" It may happen that we have a great desire for it, but if nobody takes it, we will probably give it up. Some research shows that people eat less if they are together with people who eat little and eat more if they are together with people who eat a lot. Why does this happen? In general, there are two fundamental reasons: on the one hand, if we do not know how to behave in a certain situation, which is perhaps new and unusual, we look at what others do to understand what is the appropriate behavior, and we repeat it; on the other hand, we imitate others because we identify with them because and we want to feel accepted or at least not seem strange or deviant. This is where the idea of having 3 meals a day came from. As we will see in the next chapter, however, it is *not* the best solution.

Chapter Seven

Established Intermittent Meal Plans

The recipe for living long and healthy would be to reduce protein intake: but what happens to our body with semi-fast regimes? According to Mark Mattson of the National Institute on Aging-Neuroscience, intermittent fasting generates a slight biological stress that pushes the body to reactivate its cellular defense against molecular damage. According to other experts, however, this would allow the body to detoxify, eliminating waste, toxins, and waste products.

Intermittent fasting is a flexible program and allows anyone with any kind of power to follow it. It is an effective way to lose body fat, to preserve lean mass, and to have energy throughout the fasting period.

Everyone knows what fasting is, but few people ever experience it.

Fasting is simply that time when you do not eat: usually, the longest time you do not eat is between dinner and breakfast, so that would be around 10 to 12 hours. It is no coincidence that the Anglo-Saxon countries use the word breakfast, which means "breaking a fast."

In detail, therefore, intermittent fasting (IF) is a diet that alternates phases of fasting (or underfeeding) long (from 16 to 36 hours) to feeding phases. It is simply adding a few hours to the night fast.

There are various methods: 16 hours of fasting and 8 of feeding at least 2 times a week, 16 hours of fasting and 8 of feeding every day, 24 hours of fasting 1 or 2 times a week (on the day of fasting, only one meal is eaten after 24 hours), 36 hours of fasting, and the Warrior diet (during the day, you can introduce very few calories from vegetables and/or dried fruit, and dinner only consists of just one meal).

When you follow this diet (if in good health and after consultation with your doctor), you may notice health benefits, including the decrease in body weight, decrease in blood glucose levels, increased lipolysis and fat oxidation, and decrease in stress related to food.

Is intermittent fasting good for everyone?

Intermittent fasting should not be followed by those who live the relationship with food in a nervous way, by those who cannot control the amount of food ingested, and by those who continually check the clock to know if they can start eating again.

Before making important choices from the point of view of food, you should always ask advice from an expert, primarily the family doctor—if you are in good health, and a specialist has given their consent, you can try the intermittent fasting road, perhaps starting a little at a time, grouping what you would eat during the whole day in an 8-hour band and fast the remaining 16. The goal must always be 16 hours, perhaps with the tolerance of one hour (15 to 17 hours). As always, before starting any diet or nutritional regiment, we advise you to see your doctor and discuss with him the new approach you want to take.

Why is fasting good?

As reported by Mark Mattson of the National Institute on Aging-Neuroscience, intermittent fasting provides a mild biological stress that drives the body to reactivate its cellular defense against molecular damage. Mice, for example, show higher levels of a protein that protects neurons from death. In this way, Mattson would argue that untimely fasting would remove the risk of stroke and cerebral decline, produce new neurons, and bring benefits to the whole body.

Fasting reduces inflammation, improves the immune system response, enhances the ability of cells to get rid of waste substances, slows the growth of tumors, and reduces the risk of heart disease. The thing that remains important, however, is to continue to drink lots of water. Fasting is not a low-calorie diet—a diet based on fruit or liquid. We do not consume fats, vitamins, or sugar; when you *really* fast, you do not eat anything at all.

In the body, autolysis is then started, which is essentially the process of destruction of worn out tissues. These tissues are replaced by new ones created by the same organism—in short, the body "eats itself" to regenerate itself. In addition to autolysis, fasting accelerates the cleansing of blood vessels, cells, and the environment in which they swim. So now that we have understood the basis of fasting, let's dive deeper into the topic and discover all the secrets of this modern way of eating.

Chapter Eight

Training and Fasting

For some time, there has been a total inversion with regard to the principles of weight loss and the basics of muscular anabolism.

Classic Approach

Food-induced Thermogenesis

The fundamentals of "traditional" dietetics suggest losing weight by exploiting also the specific dynamic action of food (ADS), or energy expenditure attributable to digestive, absorption, and metabolic processes.

In practice, with the same calories introduced, with increasing the division of meals, it is possible to burn more energy to process them. This allows you to reduce the amount of time "on an empty stomach" avoiding the "hunger" and keeping the metabolism speedy.

Cortisol and Thyroid Hormones

Some argue that this practice also favors the containment of an unwanted hormone, cortisol (also called "stress hormone") and maintenance of thyroid function (TSH and T3). Obviously, this system works as long as the caloric amount, the nutritional distribution, and the glycemic load-gauges of the meals are appropriate.

Preventing Catabolism

At the same time, in the context of muscle growth, it is (or was) a common opinion that to promote anabolism, it was necessary to "feed" continuously (and "as much as possible," avoiding the increase of fat) muscle fibrocells, in order to cancel any form of catabolism and promote proteosynthesis, *especially* thanks to the insulin stimulus.

What is Intermittent Fasting?

This principle is already heavily inflated and, to be sure, rather confused. It goes from the "caveman's diet," which involves a huge binge with one or two days of fasting, at the most reasoned "system 16/8" (where 16 is the hours of fasting and 8 is the hours in which 2 or 3 are consumed meals).

The cardinal principle of intermittent fasting is to create a fasting "window" (time lapse) with a duration that affects the overall caloric balance and hormone metabolism.

How Does It Work?

It seems that in conditions of food abstinence, in addition to a total insulin calm (remember that insulin is the parabolic hormone par excellence but also responsible for fat storage), there is a significant increase in another rather "interesting" hormone: l 'IGF-1 or somatomedin (some also mention an increase in testosterone).

The long deprivation of food is then responsible for the secretion of GH (somatotropin), also called "growth hormone" or, more sympathetically, "hormone of wellness." Unlike insulin, GH, while increasing hypertrophy, does not cause an adipose deposit, but the opposite! That is, it promotes the lipolysis necessary for weight loss. In practice, GH improves "all-around" body composition.

Always in bodybuilding, to increase muscle and decrease fat, it is essential to sequence the diet and training by pursuing distinctly first one and then the other goal. Today, since the intermittent fasting does result in an improvement of the body composition bilaterally (by increasing muscle mass and weight loss), it seems to be the only real solution to all problems.

Example:

Completely avoiding to cite bibliographic sources of dubious reliability (and seriousness), I will describe below the most interesting and undoubtedly best-suited variant that I could read.

First, I stress that despite using the fasting window, the remaining meals cannot be consumed freely. Moreover, to maximize the results of weight loss (and obviously those of increasing muscle mass), it is always necessary to perform the right physical activity.

The protocol differs in 3 daily meals and 1 training session with a fasting window equal to 16 hours.

- 1st meal to be eaten as soon as you rise up: a source of protein and carbohydrates with medium-low glycemic index; few fats
- 2nd meal – breakfast: complete
- Training (bodybuilding or high-intensity training)
- 3rd meal (to be done *immediately* after training) – lunch: complete

- Fasting window from 1:00 pm or 3:00 pm until the following morning.

Obviously, the system can be adapted to the lifestyle of the subject. I personally eat between 1pm and 6pm, using the mornings to do my workouts and cardio. I simply feel better not having any food in me while working, however; everyone is different though.

Chapter Nine

What Foods Can You Eat

Intermittent fasting is a diet based on the alternation of regular meals and fasting moments, with the aim of speeding up the metabolism and helping to lose weight faster. Here is an example of the benefits and the different patterns of the intermittent fasting diet.

Intermittent fasting is a diet based on the alternation of regular meals and moments of actual fasting. This type of on-off diet allows you to decide, according to different schemes, how to set the above alternation of normal meals and periods of pause from food, which would ensure a positive influence on the calorie balance and hormone metabolism, thus promoting fast weight loss and improving cardiovascular health and the immune system, in general. There are five main examples of intermittent fasting diet to choose from, in which time windows vary between fasting and normal meals, in essence.

Generally, in the examples of intermittent fasting diet, a split of the day is foreseen in two moments: a fasting phase called fast—which lasts several hours (from 12 to 19-20 hours), in which no food will be introduced with the exception of water, bitter coffee, tea and drinks without sugars—and another part called fed, in which you can eat regularly.

Intermittent Fasting: the 5 Examples of Fasting-based Diets

There are 5 main examples of a diet based on intermittent fasting. Here they are:

Intermittent Fasting or Intermittent Fasting Leangains

Devised by the athletic trainer Martin Berkhan, this method is based on scheme 16/8, i.e. the division of the day into two parts: 8 hours in which two or three meals can be consumed, and 16 hours of complete fasting.

Eat Stop Eat

This method was devised by the American nutritionist Brad Pilon, which consists of fasting for 24 hours for one or two days a week. In reality, however, in the off days, a normocaloric diet is allowed.

The Warrior Diet

This method, devised by Ori Hofmekler, provides a 4-hour fed phase—distributed between a dinner, where you can eat everything without any restriction of calories or macronutrient intake, and vegetable snacks rich in fiber and dried fruit.

The Fast Diet (or fasting every other day)

Based on the 5: 2 scheme, that is the possibility to eat regularly for 5 days a week and to make a strong calorie restriction in the other two days. In fact, in the off days, there is no actual fasting, but a maximum of 500 calories is allowed for women or 600 for men. The standard two-calorie menu should focus on a hearty breakfast—such as scrambled eggs, ham, and black tea—and a light dinner of fish or grilled chicken and vegetables. Lunch would be missed, while water and herbal teas are allowed throughout the day.

Whole Day Fasting

> It is an Eat Stop Eat with one or two days of complete fasting, unlike the diet devised by Pilon. The good news is that in the other 5/6 days you can eat ad libitum (as you desire).

Intermittent fasting: What to Eat?

But what to eat in the fed phases of the various intermittent fasting diets?

Let us consider as the first example the most frequent type of intermittent fasting, which concentrates the fed phase in 8 hours, followed by a 16-hour fast. Here is a recommended-type menu:

Breakfast
Green tea, bitter coffee or herbal tea without sugar, water at will. (This phase is still fasting, considering that these drinks can be consumed safely even in the hours of fasting.)

Lunch (from 12 onwards)
Pasta with pesto, mixed vegetables with a spoon of oil, a fruit. (From here begins the fed phase, where you can have meals for the next 8 hours.)

Snack (from 16)
Dried fruit 15g, a fruit, 50g of rice or corn cakes

Dinner (at 19)
Baked cod, rye bread, mixed vegetables seasoned with a tablespoon of oil, a glass (125 mL) of wine. (Remember to stop the fed phase after 8 hours from the start of your first meal, breakfast excluded.)

This type of menu can also be followed for the 4 hours of fed Warrior Diet, to which is added the possibility of snacks based on vegetables rich in fiber and nuts—as well as for the two-day low-calorie diet Eat Stop Eat but trying to limit the doses, as they are days of reduction and semi-fasting to which they follow 5-6 wherein you can eat freely.

For the Whole Day Fasting Diet, there is no need for any indication, as unlike the previous ones where the fast is partial or relegated to some moments of the day, there are two days of absolute fasting per week, where you are only allowed to drink water, tea, and unsweetened drinks. For the others 5 days, there is no restriction.

Fast diet: what to eat in the 5:2 diet

Regarding the Fast diet, or diet every other day, based on the scheme 5:2, i.e. 5 days at full speed and 2 days at caloric restriction, the standard menu for the two days off provides a balance shared between an abundant breakfast and a light dinner that prefers protein foods.

Breakfast
Scrambled eggs, a thin slice of ham, and black tea

Dinner
Fish, chicken, and vegetables (all preferably grilled)
Water, herbal teas, or unsweetened green or black tea at will

Intermittent Fasting: When to Avoid It?

Although it is not such a drastic diet, intermittent fasting is not suitable for everyone. It is, in fact, not recommended for people suffering from diabetes, hypoglycemia, and cortisol imbalance.

It is also best to avoid it if you are subject to chronic fatigue or being pregnant or breastfeeding.

What to Eat in Intermittent Fasting: Guidelines

To make the most of your calorie intake on a day of fasting:

1) Choose more protein meals that help you feel full longer. Because proteins have enough calories, you cannot take unlimited amounts to reach the maximum limit set by your fasting day, which is 500 calories. However, you can still make proteins the main source of calories.

2) Fill the dish with low-calorie vegetables. They give a sense of satiety, are tasty, and are good for the health. Cook with steam, bake with a teaspoon of oil, or sauté in the pan. Then, add some spices or flavorings to prepare a tasty meal. You can also choose to eat raw salad.

3) Keep the carbohydrates to a minimum: they are rich in calories and make you feel hungry quickly. Among the high-carbohydrate foods, you should avoid potatoes, sweet potatoes, pasta, rice, bread, some fruits (bananas, grapes, melons, prunes, raisins, dates, and other nuts), breakfast cereals, fruit juices, corn-sole-panicle/sweet corn, and anything containing sugar or other syrups.

4) Do not be afraid of fat: although fat is rich in calories, it helps you feel full. Include small amounts of fat in the fasting meal.

Although the recommended caloric intake is 500 calories for women and 600 calories for men, it is not necessary to be really so stiff—but it will be necessary to weigh or measure at least the high-calorie ingredients in your recipes and calculate the calories to avoid overeating the allowed threshold.

A prepared meal can be a solution without too many problems. As with home-cooked meals, look for options that are low in carbohydrates and sugars and rich in protein and vegetables.

What to eat after fasting?

Intermittent fasting is the best way to eat for food lovers! In the days of not fasting, you are free to eat whatever you want, generally speaking.

Although, of course, if you want to lose weight, maybe you'll have to limit yourself to eating whatever you want. **Additionally, as strange as it may seem, the days where you do not fast probably will help you reduce your appetite instead of increasing it.**

You may find that you are not very hungry the day after fasting. You do not need to eat much if you do not want to. It is advisable, instead, to wait to feel the stimulus of hunger before eating on a day when you are not fasting.

Your tastes can change so as to no longer feel the desire for sweet and sugary foods.

You will understand hunger better, and you will feel less the desire to eat snacks. Then, you can develop the ability to wait for meals without worrying about when it will be time to eat.

This kind of changes will not happen immediately: your hunger on non-fasting days can vary greatly. You may find that you are really hungry and eat a lot on the days when you do not fast.

Many people experience this in the early days.

Do not worry if this happens; focus only on following your scheduled fasts.

After 6 weeks of fasting, if you still have hunger problems and cannot limit yourself to food and therefore are not losing weight, you may decide to change the method of fasting or make other changes. You should aim to eat normally on days when you are not fasting.

The joy of intermittent fasting is that you can spend most of your free time on food anxiety while controlling your weight and living healthily.

Some people limit their calories on days when they do not fast in an attempt to accelerate weight loss. Although this may work in the short term, it's probably not a good idea in the long run.

If you do not have your normal feeding days, you will probably feel deprived of your favorite foods and develop "diet fatigue."

If intermittent fasting has to become your way of life, it is important that you do it sustainably for a long time.

Chapter Ten

Sample Meal Ideas

Intermittent Fasting Food Plan

The intermittent fasting food plan by Ori Hofmekler is based on a very simple and intuitive structure:

Phase 1 - Under Power (for about 20 hours)

> During the first part of the day, few foods are allowed—mostly of plant origin, such as seeds and simple proteins, i.e. all foods that are not very demanding for our digestive system. This is intended to facilitate detoxification of the body.
>
> The prolonged (but controlled) state of under-feeding triggers physiological processes such as increased insulin sensitivity and increased production of anabolic hormones to counteract the state of "resource shortage" and to make the most of the few present.

Phase 2 – Supercharging (for the remaining 4 hours)

> After Phase 1, the body finds itself *emptied* of resources and in a condition of maximum sensitivity to nourishment.
>
> This particular condition makes sure that a large amount of nutrients introduced during supercharging is not lost or "stored" as fat (also due to the low level of insulin).

During this phase, there is no particular constraint on the type of food to be taken or its quantity.

Of course, taking on a diet like this also requires a team of specialists to follow you on the way, since you must not forget that you are a unique biological entity, and as such you will have individual responses that will need specific adjustments to allow optimization of the diet without incurring problems of any kind.

If some types of food programs are intuitive because they involve phases of total fasting in phases in which you can eat anything, in other cases indications are needed.

Take for example the leangains diet which, as mentioned, provides a fed phase of 8 hours, and a fast phase of 16 hours.

At breakfast and throughout the day you can give yourself green tea, bitter coffee, unsweetened teas, water.

At lunch, instead, after 12, you can eat pasta with pesto, mixed vegetables with a tablespoon of oil, fruit. (From here begins the fed phase, where you can have meals for the next 8 hours)

From 4 pm, you can have a snack with 15 g of dried fruit, a fruit and 50 g of rice or corn cakes.

At dinner, after 7 pm, the program includes baked cod, rye or wholemeal bread, mixed vegetables seasoned with a tablespoon of oil, a glass of wine. It is important to stop the fed phase, after 8 hours from the start of the first meal, excluding breakfast.

The fast diet consists of 5 days in which you eat regularly and 2 days of caloric restriction. In these 2 days the consumption of protein foods is recommended. At breakfast, you can eat for example, scrambled eggs, ham and tea; for dinner, instead, chicken, fish and grilled vegetables.

The most frequent type of intermittent fasting is leangains, which concentrates the fed phase in 8 hours, followed by a 16-hour fast. Below we propose an example of a menu, which must however be modified according to the different needs:

Breakfast: green tea, bitter coffee or herbal tea without sugar, water at will. This phase is still fasting;

Lunch: wholemeal pasta, mixed vegetables with a tablespoon of oil, a fruit. From here begins the fed phase;

Snack: dried fruit, a fruit, rice cakes or corn or a low-fat yogurt;

Dinner: meat and lean fish baked or grilled, tofu or seitan, rye or wholemeal bread, mixed vegetables seasoned with a tablespoon of oil. This is the last phase of fed.

It is important to stop the fed phase after 8 hours from the start of your first meal (breakfast excluded since you consume only liquids). So, for example, if you eat lunch at 12 you can eat until 8pm.

Additional Resources

Here is a collection of studies that can help you better understand the concepts discussed in the book:

https://www.ncbi.nlm.nih.gov/pmc/articles/PMC3680567/

https://www.ncbi.nlm.nih.gov/pmc/articles/PMC4403246/

https://www.health.harvard.edu/blog/intermittent-fasting-surprising-update-2018062914156

https://newatlas.com/intermittent-fasting-16-8-diet-study-science/55105/

https://newatlas.com/intermittent-fasting-causes-diabetes-debate/54685/

https://www.healthline.com/nutrition/intermittent-fasting-guide

https://www.businessinsider.com/intermittent-fasting-diet-health-benefits-weight-loss-2018-6

https://www.johnshopkinshealthreview.com/issues/spring-summer-2016/articles/are-there-any-proven-benefits-to-fasting

https://sciencebasedmedicine.org/intermittent-fasting/

https://thedoctorweighsin.com/what-science-has-to-say-about-intermittent-fasting/

https://www.popsci.com/intermittent-fasting-science

Conclusion

The next step is to stop reading and to start doing whatever it is that you need to do in order to ensure that you are able to create amazing intermittent fasting recipes and dishes. If you find that you still need help getting started, you will likely have better results by creating a schedule that you hope to follow—including strict deadlines for various parts of the tasks as well as the overall completion of your preparations.

Studies show that complex tasks that are broken down into individual pieces, including individual deadlines, have a much greater chance of being completed when compared to something that has a general need of being completed but no real timetable for doing so. Even if it seems silly, go ahead and set your own deadlines for completion—complete with indicators of success and failure. After you have successfully completed all your required preparations, you will be glad you did. For example, you can think about practicing one new intermittent fasting food habit every day, before becoming a general master of the diet. It is your choice, and it is the beauty of dieting and cooking.

Once you have tried the same recipe many times, it is the right moment to invite your friends and ask them to try the intermittent fasting diet—they are going to love it and, best of all, see incredible results with it.

Made in the
USA
Monee, IL